"BONE GRAFTING IN ORAL IMPLANTOLOGY"
Techniques & Clinical Applications

Original Title: Injertos Óseos en Implantología
Técnicas y Aplicaciones Clínicas
by Federico Hernández Alfaro
MD, DDS, PhD, FEBOMS

Bone Grafting in Oral Implantology
Techniques and Clinical Applications

quintessence
books

© Federico Hernández Alfaro
© 2006 Quintessence Publishing Co.Ltd. (UK)

ISBN: 1-85097-103-X

Printed in Spain

Bone Grafting in Oral
Implantology
Techniques and Clinical Applications

EDITOR

FEDERICO HERNANDEZ ALFARO,
MD, DDS, PhD, FEBOMS

Clinical Professor, Oral and Maxillofacial Surgery
& Coordinator Program in Oral Implantology,
Universitat Internacional de Catalunya,
Barcelona, Spain

Chief, Department of Oral and Maxillofacial Surgery,
Hospital General de Catalunya & Teknon Medical Center,
Barcelona, Spain

Quintessence Publishing Co.Ltd.
London, Berlin, Chicago, Tokyo, Barcelona, Beijing, Istanbul, Milan,
Moscow, Mumbai, Paris, Prague, São Paulo, Seoul, Warsaw

CONTRIBUTORS

CARLOS ARRANZ, MD
Associate Professor, Oral and Maxillofacial Surgery, Universitat Internacional de Catalunya, Barcelona, Spain
Staff, Department of Oral and Maxillofacial Surgery Teknon Medical Center, Barcelona, Spain

MARIA JOSE BIOSCA, MD, DDS
Associate Professor, Oral and Maxillofacial Surgery, Universitat Internacional de Catalunya, Barcelona, Spain
Staff, Department of Oral and Maxillofacial Surgery, Hospital General de Catalunya & Teknon Medical Center, Barcelona, Spain

ELOY GARCIA, MD, FEBOMS
Staff, Department of Oral and Maxillofacial Surgery, Hospital Clinic & Teknon Medical Center, Barcelona, Spain

JAVIER GIMENO, MD
Associate Professor, Oral and Maxillofacial Surgery, Universitat Internacional de Catalunya, Barcelona, Spain
Staff, Department of Oral and Maxillofacial Surgery, Hospital General de Catalunya & Teknon Medical Center, Barcelona, Spain

CARLOS MARTI, MD
Associate Professor, Oral and Maxillofacial Surgery, Universitat Internacional de Catalunya, Barcelona, Spain
Staff, Department of Oral and Maxillofacial Surgery, Hospital General de Catalunya & Teknon Medical Center, Barcelona, Spain

ACKNOWLEDGMENTS

The authors are indebted to Laura García Arana, MD, for her assistance in preparing the manuscript.
We also want to thank Emilio González Matheu, MD, DDS, and Luis Aulló for their superb drawings.

FOREWORD

Rehabilitation of the lost alveolar bone is today inherent in preprosthetic implantology. Optimal implant positioning is essential to achieve normal anatomical relationships within the oral cavity.

Oral and maxillofacial surgery techniques have been incorporated into routine implant practice to restore normal anatomy, thus allowing ideal implant positioning.

This book clearly presents, in an orderly way, different alternatives for bone harvesting. Both intra- and extraoral sources have been analysed thoroughly, using a very practical approach. The description of varied clinical applications in each chapter is extremely useful for the clinician facing multiple reconstructive situations in the preprosthetic surgical practice.

The authors are to be commended for their systematic and detailed description of all the harvesting techniques. It is noteworthy that a vast array of clinical examples has been incorporated for each harvesting site. This proves the fact that surgeons must have competence in all harvesting techniques. In this way optimally tailored solutions can be found for a specific clinical case.

Dr. Hernández Alfaro and his co-authors have established a standard in preprosthetic bone surgery and convey it in the clearest possible terms. In summary, this book may be relied on as an emminently practical guide to sound clinical practice.

Carlos Navarro-Vila
Full Professor of Maxillofacial Surgery
Medical School
Universidad Complutense de Madrid

Chief Department Oral and Maxillofacial Surgery
Hospital Gregorio Marañon
Madrid, Spain

PREFACE

Bone reconstruction in implantology constitutes a challenge for the surgeon. The time when lack of bone in the oral region constituted a contraindication for implant therapy are over.

Oral and maxillofacial surgery techniques allow harvesting of bone from different locations in the body in order to reconstruct defective areas in the oral region. Contemporary implant prosthetics have increased aesthetic and functional demands, and normalisation of alveolar architecture must be a goal.

This book is a direct consequence of our clinical activity for the past 12 years. Our postgraduate students have been a stimulus in their desire to have a comprehensive manual for their daily practice. On the other hand, our courses on the subject have obliged us to compile and systematically organise our clinical material. Our approach overall has been pragmatic. The goal is to allow surgeons involved in implant therapy to incorporate different procedures for oral bone reconstruction.

When designing the book, we decided that organising it by donor sites could facilitate understanding of the pros and cons of each of them, still giving a clear view of all the different indications. We strongly believe that when approaching advanced oral reconstruction one has to know all the sources for autogenous bone grafts in order to choose the best option for a given defect.

We will show how similar clinical situations can be managed with different strategies and donor sites.

In each chapter a brief anatomical review of the site is followed by a thorough description of the harvesting technique. The third part of each chapter is devoted to clinical applications of a given graft, followed by a list of potential complications of the harvesting technique. Finally, a bibliography is provided.

I am very grateful to Drs. Arranz, Biosca, García, Giméno and Martí for their contribution to the book. It has been a pleasure to share with them my clinical as well as academic activity for the past 12 years.

Federico Hernández Alfaro
MD, DDS, PhD, FEBOMS

CONTENTS

7

Chapter 1

Biology of Bone Grafting

Why Bone Grafts?

The need for bone grafting reflects the fact that edentulous situations are very often associated with variable degrees of bone resorption. The remodelling process that will eventually lead to different degrees of alveolar atrophy starts the very first day after tooth removal or avulsion (Fig 1-1 a-m).

A graft is a portion of a tissue or an organ that, after removal from its origin or 'donor' site, is positioned or inserted at a different place or recipient site with the objective of reinforcing the existing tissues and/or correcting a structural defect. The aim is for the graft to eventually receive nutrition from the host.

Autografts are transplants from one region to another in the same individual. Therefore no histocompatibility issues have to be considered.[1]

Bone grafts can remain functional from a structural point of view even when the original cell population does not persist. The bony matrix eventually becomes repopulated by invading cells from the host in a process known as 'creeping substitution'. This does not work for skin or mucous membrane, for which viability of the original cell population is essential for success of the graft.[2]

Bone Autografts

Bone is probably the most frequently transplanted tissue in the body. It can be used to treat or repair defects resulting from atrophy, injury, congenital malformations or neoplasms.

Reconstruction of bone defects has been a challenge for oral and maxillofacial surgeons. On the other hand, knowledge of bone repair and graft behaviour has allowed the design of protocols for harvesting, preserving and eventually inserting the grafts.

Autogenous bone has been the only source of osteogenic cells to date and thus is considered the gold standard for oral reconstruction.

9

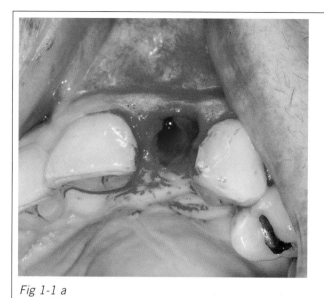

Fig 1-1 a

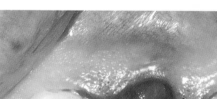

Fig 1-1 (a-c) Removal of a failed upper lateral leaves a three-wall defect in the socket due to resorption of the vestibular wall. Note how probing reveals a 9mm vertical defect. If reconstruction of the alveolus is not undertaken future implant stability and, most importantly, aesthetics will be severely compromised.

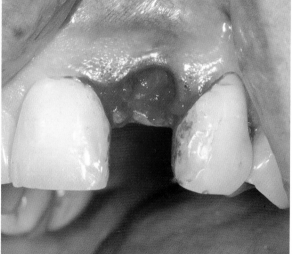

Fig 1-1 c

Fig 1-1 b

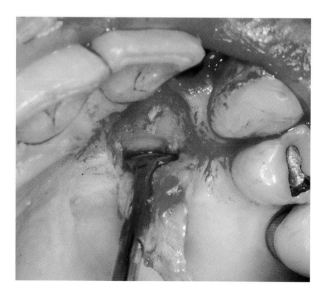

Fig 1-1 (d) A palatal posteriorly pedicled flap is developed, uncovering the palatal vault in the vicinity.

Fig 1-1 (e-g) A trephine 6mm in diameter is used to harvest a cylinder of cortical bone. The trephine acts parallel to the neighbouring roots.

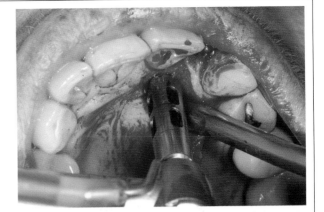

Fig 1-1 e

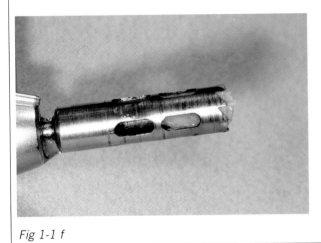

Fig 1-1 f

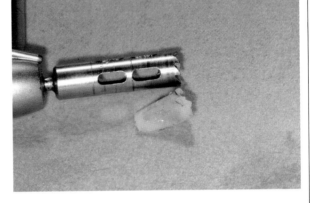

Fig 1-1 g

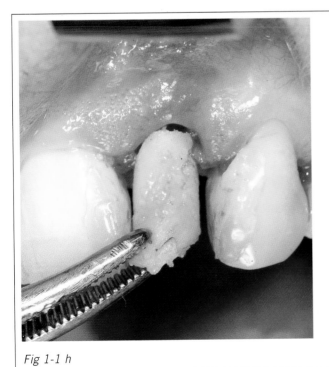

Fig 1-1 h

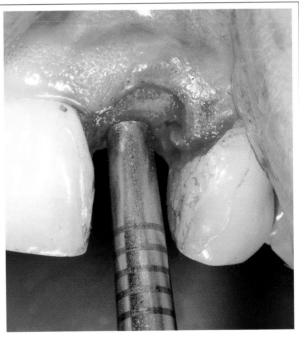

Fig 1-1 i

Fig 1-1 (h, i) With the aid of a flat-ended osteotome the graft is impacted in the socket.

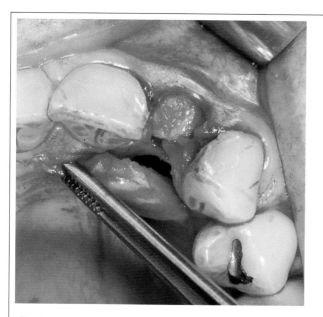

Fig 1-1 j

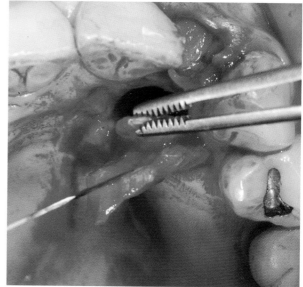

Fig 1-1 k

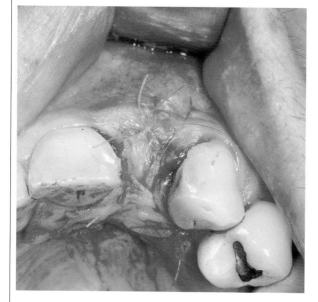

Fig 1-1 l

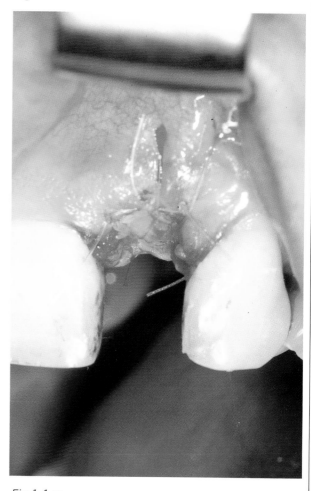

Fig 1-1 (j, m) A split-thickness palatal flap is tailored and rotated to protect the reconstruction. This connective tissue flap will eventually transform into keratinised mucosa.

Fig 1-1 m

Healing of Bone Grafts

Incorporation of the grafts happens in concert with a process of initial remodelling and resorption, which is associated with a loss of bone volume. The amount and rate of resorption depends on many factors, such as dimensions of the bone graft, the quality of bone, the quality of the recipient site, biomechanical properties and fixation to the surrounding bone (Fig 1-2 a, b).[3]

Reviewing the stages of revascularisation and healing of bone grafts is essential to understand their behaviour and outcome.

When the bone graft is first placed in the area the cortical portion of the bone is avascular and has very few viable cells on its surface. This bone graft eventually becomes replaced by host bone.

During this substitution, a vascular sequence follows. The area surrounding the bone graft becomes hypervascular. The bone graft itself elicits proliferation of angioblasts and small capillaries in the early stages. This angioblastic proliferation occurs within the first week of grafting. These blood vessels carry the elements for osteogenic bone formation and replacement. Osteoclasts are present at this early stage, resorbing the bone at the periphery of the graft. The bone graft is gradually replaced while new bone is laid down at the periphery and inside. The graft is replaced in a period that lasts between three and six months. When this occurs the hypervascularity gradually disappears.[4]

There is a histological response running parallel to the vascular one. Granulation tissue with fibroblastic and angioblastic proliferation is followed by proliferation of immature osteoid tissue at the periphery of the graft. After the osteoid is replaced by mature bone there is no evidence of the grafted avascular bone graft.[5]

Graft healing occurs in one of three ways: osteogenesis, osteoinduction or osteoconduction. The proportions of these processes in each case depend largely on the type of graft and conditions of the host site.[6]

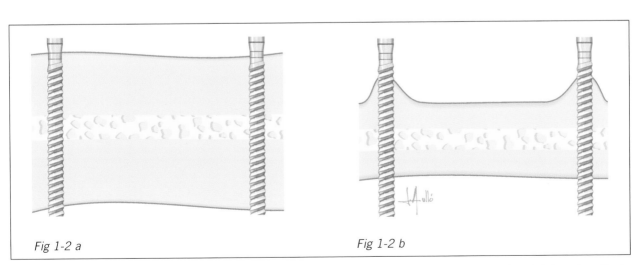

Fig 1-2 a

Fig 1-2 b

Fig 1-2 (a, b) Graft resorption depends largely on the type of bone (for instance, embryologic origin) and methods of fixation.

Osteogenesis occurs when the graft itself supplies viable osteoblasts (osteogenic cells) as the source of new bone. It is well known that bone sources (for instance, the iliac crest) with high proportions of marrow have better osteogenic properties due to an increased number of undifferentiated cells. Osteoinduction occurs when the graft 'activates' the surrounding host tissues, through signalling factors, to stimulate osteoclastic activity and new bone formation. Osteoinduction has classically been related to autologous fresh bone transplants. More recently, recombinant bone morphogenetic proteins (rh BMP) have been developed to induce bone formation.[7] Finally, osteoconduction occurs when undifferentiated mesenchymal cells invade the graft, which acts as a scaffold or physical matrix. This matrix allows deposition of new bone. The graft material should allow bone to form without impeding this process.[8]

During the healing phase of a graft there is competition between bone-forming cells and soft tissue-forming cells to fill the defect.

As mentioned earlier, the gold standard for bone reconstruction is the fresh autograft. Among different autologous sources, cancellous bone from the iliac crest has been considered the reference source, due to its enhanced osteogenic properties.[9]

Types of Grafts

Bone grafts can be classified according to the structure, source and immune response, and embryological origin.

Bone grafts classified according to the structure (Fig 1-3 a, b) include:
- Cortical - Skull, chin and body of mandible.
- Cancellous - Inner tibia or iliac crest.
- Cortico-cancellous or composite - Blocks from the iliac crest.

Bone grafts classified according to source and immune response include:
- Autograft or autologous.
- Allograft - From a different human.

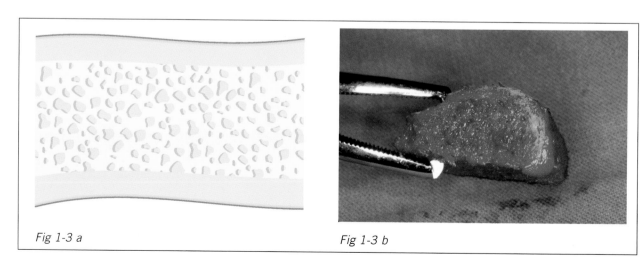

Fig 1-3 a

Fig 1-3 b

Fig 1-3 (a, b) The proportion of cancellous/cortical bone varies between different donor sites. Iliac crest blocks have high amounts of cancellous bone and a rather thin cortical layer.

- Xenograft - From another living being.
- Alloplast or synthetic.

Bone grafts classified according to embryological origin include:

- Membranous - Originated from mesenchymal cells (for instance, all the bone located in the craniofacial skeleton).
- Enchondral - Originated from ectomesenchymal cells (for instance, iliac crest, tibia).

Cancellous Bone

This is rich in osteogenic cells, especially those from the iliac crest. If adequate manipulation of the graft is completed, osteoblasts may survive more than three hours. Surviving cells tend to be close to the recipient surface and resist anoxia due to diffusion mechanisms. If the host site has been adequately prepared, early revascularisation may be present as soon as 48 hours after grafting.

Drawbacks of cancellous bone include lack of structural rigidity, which complicates 3D reconstructions, and less resistance to resorption.

The main sources for cancellous bone are iliac crest and tibia. Minor amounts can be found in the chin and tuberosity.

Cortical Bone

This type of bone is highly osteoconductive due to the Haversian system and thus more resistant to resorption, which is useful when structural rigidity is an issue. It is however deficient in osteogenic cells (Fig 1-4 a).

Cortical bone can be harvested in large quantities from the parietal bones. The problem of medium-sized defects can be solved with blocks from the chin, and from the body and ramus of the mandible (Fig 1-4 b). The zygomatic buttress is the more suitable for small defects or dehiscences.

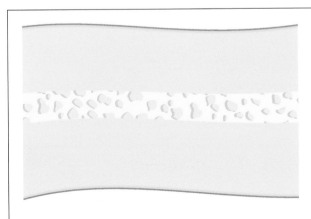

Fig 1-4 a

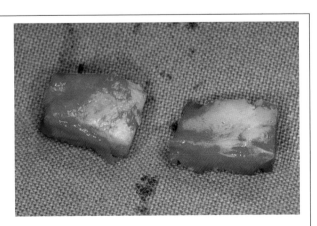

Fig 1-4 b

Fig 1-4 (a, b) Chin grafts are mainly cortical with scarce proportions of cancellous bone.

References

1   Block MS, Kent JN. Sinus augmentation for dental implants: The use of autogenous bone. J Oral Maxillofac Surg 1997;55:1281-1286.

2   Burwell RG. Osteogenesis in cancellous bone grafts: Considered in terms of cellular changes, basic mechanisms and the perspective of growth control and its possible aberrations. Clin Orthop 1965;40:35.

3   Fonseca RJ, Clark PJ, Burkes EJ Jr, Baker RD. Revascularization and healing of onlay particulate autologous bone grafts in primates. J Oral Maxillofac Surg 1980;38:572-577.

4   Stroud SW, Fonseca RJ, Sanders GW, Burkes EJ Jr. Healing of interpositional autologous bone grafts after total maxillary osteotomy. J Oral Surg 1980;38:878-885.

5   Hollinger JO, Wong MEK. The integrated processes of hard tissue regeneration with special emphasis on fracture healing. Oral Surg Oral Med Oral Pathol 1996;82:594.

6   Moy PK. Clinical experience with osseous site development using autogenous bone, bone graft substitutes and membrane barriers. Oral Maxillofac Surg Clin North Am 2001;13:493-509.

7   Wozney J. The bone morphogenetic protein family and osteogenesis. Mol Reprod Develop 1992;32:160-166.

8   Moy P. Clinical experience with osseous site development using autogenous bone, bone substitutes and membrane barriers. Oral Maxillofac Surg Clin North Am 2001;13:493-509.

9   Collins M, James DR, Mars M. Alveolar bone grafting: A review of 115 patients. Eur J Orthod 1998;20:115-120.

General Principles of Bone Grafting

Management of Bone Grafts

Preservation

One of the main goals when harvesting bone grafts is preservation of the highest possible number of living osteoblasts.

Sterility must be preserved from removal of the graft until its delivery at the recipient site.

Once removed it can be kept enveloped in moist gauze. This can be soaked with isotonic serum or, even better, with autologous blood or platelet-rich plasma (PRP) (Fig 2-1 a, b). Soaking the graft in saline may accelerate cell lysis. Some authors recommend embedding the graft with antibiotics to protect it until revascularisation takes place.

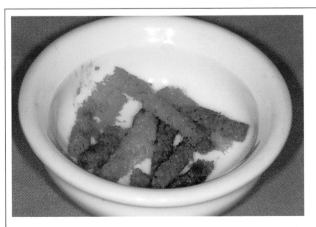
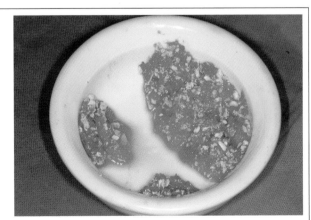

Fig 2-1 a *Fig 2-1 b*

Fig 2-1 (a, b) Cancellous bone from the tibia before and after mixture with PRP and bovine anorganic bone to facilitate handling and delay resorption respectively.

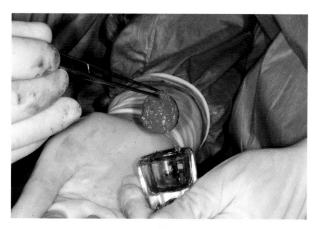

Fig 2-2 Bone 'croquette' ready to be delivered at the recipient site.

For better handling of cancellous or particulated grafts we strongly recommend the use of PRP as a 'biological' carrier. This mixture gives stability to the graft and facilitates manipulation and delivery to the recipient site. Through the use of PRP as a 'carrier', the transport and adaptation of particulated grafts has become much easier (Fig 2-2).

Cortical and composite blocks need to be adequately adapted and fixed to the recipient site in order to allow incorporation. Big grafts from the iliac crest or the calvarium usually need to be cut into different pieces before adaptation.

Trimming

In most instances grafts need to be adapted to the defective area. The proportion of cortical bone (rigidity) of the graft usually correlates with the difficulty in adaptation to the host site.

Cancellous bone is usually condensed and applied with the aid of sterile syringes or bone carriers into a cavity or space (for instance, maxillary sinus).

Before the harvesting procedure it is of the utmost importance to determine accurately the shape and size of grafts needed in order to limit morbidity and avoid wasting material (Fig 2-3 a, b)

Saws, burs and rongeurs are necessary to trim the blocks, and if particulated bone is needed for a specific reconstruction it might also be necessary to grind cortical blocks with a bone mill.

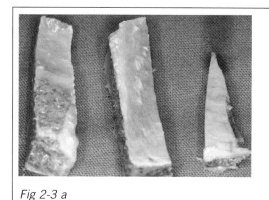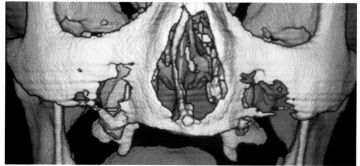

Fig 2-3 a

Fig 2-3 b

Fig 2-3 (a, b) Accurate planning of bone grafting requires determination of the volume needed through a CT scan. A severe atrophy of the maxilla is to be reconstructed with cortico-cancellous blocks from the iliac crest. Determination of the actual needs should be as accurate as possible to minimise morbidity.

Recipient site

Preparation of the recipient site includes adequate periosteal elevation and peeling of all fibrous remnants inserted in or adherent to the bone.

To 'activate' the recipient bed we recommend performing small perforations in the cortex with a fissure bur. This seems to facilitate vascular and tissue in-growth from the medullary area in the host bone into the graft.

Fixation

Fixation of the graft, in cases in which it is in the form of a block, is done with miniscrews. The number of screws needed to fix a graft rigidly remains the subject of controversy.

In most cases a single screw will suffice to stabilise a small or medium-sized block (Fig 2-4 a-d). Big blocks, especially those from the iliac crest, which often require 'flexible' adaptation, may need two or more screws to achieve perfect stabilisation of the graft (Fig 2-5 a-c).

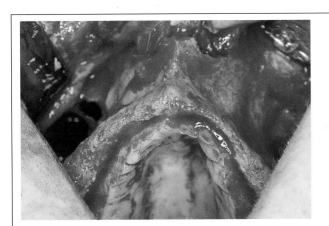

Fig 2-4 a

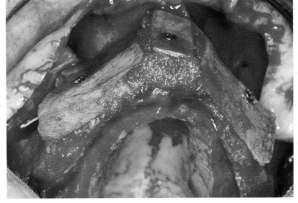

Fig 2-4 b

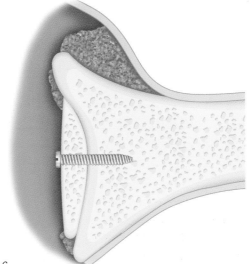

Fig 2-4 (a-c) Severe AP atrophy of the maxilla reconstructed with blocks from the iliac crest. Note how each block is held in place with a single screw.

Fig 2-4 c

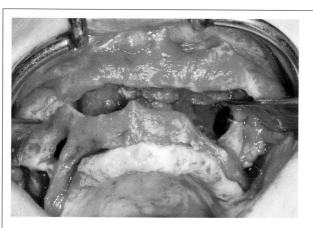

Fig 2-4 (d) A long calvarial graft fixed to posterior mandible with a single compression screw.

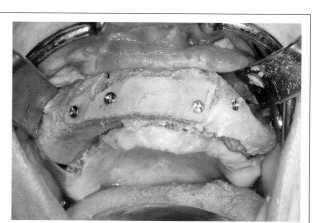

Fig 2-5 a

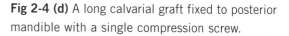

Fig 2-5 b

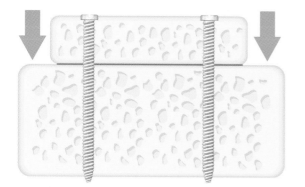

Fig 2-5 c

Fig 2-5 (a-c) There are situations where long blocks have to be bent and adapted to the convex shape of the anterior maxilla. This is about the only indication for multiple screw fixation of a graft. Cortico-cancellous blocks from the iliac crest are prone to bending due to the thin and elastic cortex.

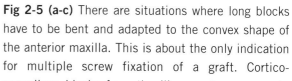

The screws should act in a compression fashion - that is, the hole in the graft should be bigger than the screw. This way the shaft of the screw will circulate freely through the graft and the head of the screw will compress the block against the recipient site.

Screws with a diameter of 1.5mm or 2.0mm are currently used for graft fixation.

Rigid fixation is mandatory for bone graft survival, and compression screws are the best way to achieve it. There are instances where screw fixation is not possible and either wire or suture fixation can be applied so that the graft is protected from load during the healing period (Fig 2-6 a, b, c).

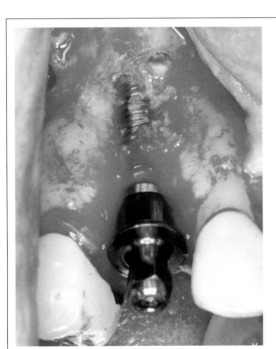

Fig 2-6 a

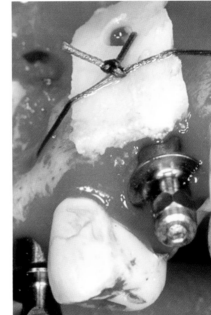

Fig 2-6 b

Fig 2-6 (a-c) Simultaneous onlay grafting and fixture insertion. It is impossible to place a screw in order to fix the veneer graft. Thus a trans-crestal resorbable 4/0 suture is used to secure the block in place. This kind of approach can be taken only in situations where the graft is protected from tensions or pressure.

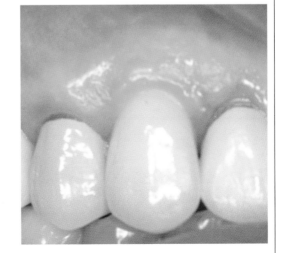

Fig 2-6 c

Soft-tissue coverage

Independent of the type of graft used and the area reconstructed, watertight closure of the reconstruction is mandatory and flap design is of the outmost importance for all grafting procedures. Preserving blood supply, keeping the periosteum intact and avoiding tears through the mucosa will add protection to the reconstruction. Quite often the increase of volume associated with bone grafting will render the surrounding soft tissue insufficient to cover it. In these situations it is advisable to perform relieving incisions in the periosteum, which should be parallel to the borders of the flaps. Periosteal release will allow extra stretching of the flaps and advancement without tension. Some authors advocate the use of PRP to enhance soft-tissue healing.

Re-entry

On limited occasions, bone grafting and fixture insertion is completed simultaneously. In these instances fixation screws can be left in place or removed, depending on how they interact with the covering tissues.

When fixture installation is done at a later stage than the bone grafting procedure we often find that the fixation screws are in the way of fixture insertion. In these cases the screws should be removed, preserving mucoperiosteal insertions and, when possible, in a flapless fashion (Fig 2-7 a-h).

22

Fig 2-7 (a-h) Re-entry for fixture insertion in cases of bone grafting should minimise mucoperiosteal stripping to reduce trauma and protect the reconstructed area. When possible we recommend a transmucous flapless approach to remove the fixation screw.

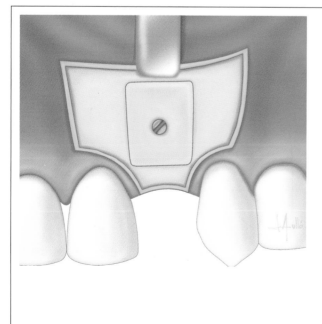

Fig 2-7 a

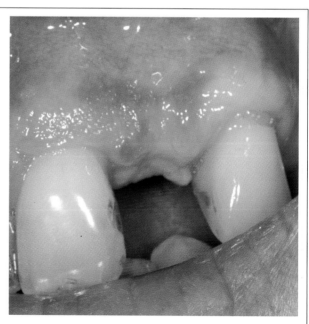

Fig 2-7 b

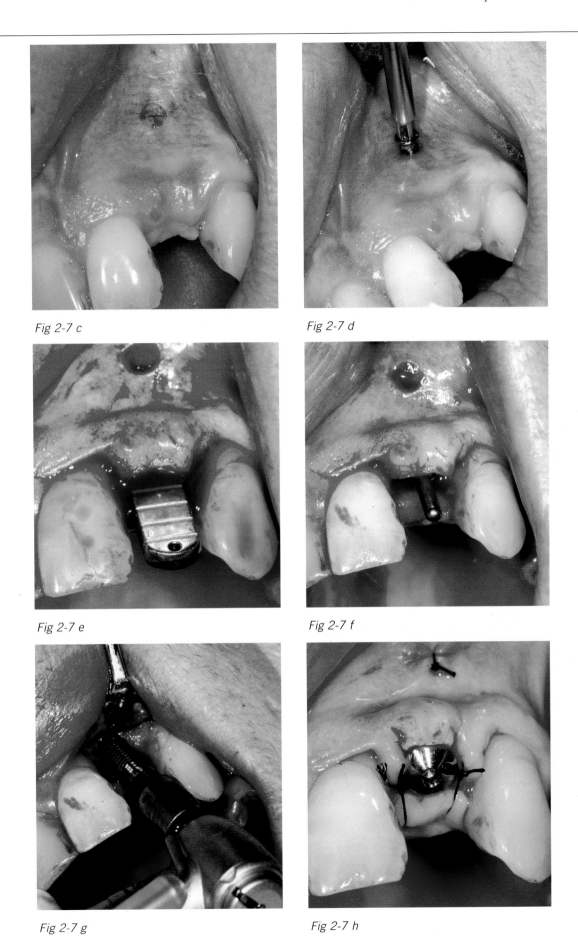

Fig 2-7 c

Fig 2-7 d

Fig 2-7 e

Fig 2-7 f

Fig 2-7 g

Fig 2-7 h

Harvesting and Fixation Instruments

Bone grafting requires a specific armamentarium that varies according to the donor site (Fig 2-8).

Intraoral Harvesting

There is a specific armamentarium for bone harvesting, depending on the donor site.

General oral surgery instruments are common to any oral surgery procedure.

Bone-cutting instruments

The ideal bone cutter should be fast, easy to handle and as atraumatic as possible.

- Saws (reciprocating and oscillating) are ideal in cases where thin cuts are necessary. The drawbacks are difficulties in reaching certain areas of the oral cavity, cost and the fact that thin cuts do not allow chisels to get in.

- Fissure burs are used for corticotomies and round lab burs for graft remodelling. They are very effective, easy to handle and cheap.
- Discs are dangerous unless guarded. They can easily 'run' into the soft tissues causing lacerations. They are the 'cheap' alternative to saws.
- Rongeurs are excellent for harvesting and/or cutting bone from the tuberosity area. They bite soft bone very atraumatically.
- Chisels are good as osteotomes in the maxilla. They should not be used in the mandible - at least not maleted - to avoid trauma to the temporomandibular joint. They are effective in 'elevating' bone grafts once corticotomes have been completed.

Bone-milling devices

There are several companies producing such instruments. A sharp bone rongeur can be a good substitute.

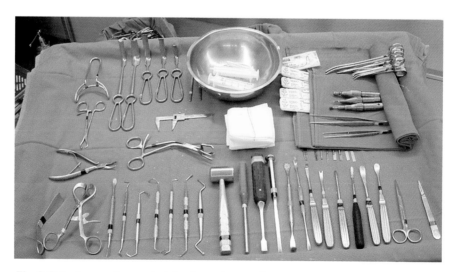

Fig 2-8 Instruments needed for bone harvesting vary between different donor sites. It is practical to standardise the various items needed for each procedure.

Extraoral Harvesting

Calvarial (parietal)

Orthostatic tissue retractors keep the edges of the incision away.

Curved osteotomes dislodge the graft in an angled fashion.

Tibia

Manually or automatically driven trephines are useful to perform the small round ostectomy that allows access to the tibial methaphysis.

Curettes (straight and curved) are used to dislodge cancellous bone from the medullary cavity.

Bone filters are used to remove the loose particles of bone.

Iliac crest

Orthopaedic retractors (Taylor, Hoffman) are used to separate the abdominal contents.

Larger chisels, blades and curettes are also needed.

Chapter 3

Symphysis (Chin)

The mandibular symphysis also known as the chin or 'menton' has been previously reported in the literature as a donor site in preprosthetic reconstruction of the atrophic maxilla and mandible.[1-10]

Clinical studies on the comparison of chin grafts with iliac crest or rib grafts in the reconstruction of alveolar clefts reveal only minimal complications at the mandibular donor site and significantly less resorption associated with chin grafts.[11]

Experimental evidence also suggests that intramembranous bone grafts maintain more volume and show less resorption than endochondral grafts.[12,13] This is probably due to the faster revascularisation and slower resorption of the membranous bone.[14,15]

To avoid excessive resorption of the chin graft, we recommend fixture installation no later than three months after graft placement. In some instances graft and implant placement can be done simultaneously if stability of both is guaranteed.[16,17]

Compared with other intraoral sites, such as tuberosity, zygoma, palate, and coronoid process, the symphyseal region can provide higher quantities of bone. Other advantages of chin grafts include diminished postoperative morbidity, reduced or eliminated hospital stay, which decreases costs, minimal postoperative discomfort, no alteration in ambulation, and avoidance of cutaneous scars.[3] The chin graft is reliable and can be harvested in an office setting with low morbidity and high patient acceptance.

Surgical Anatomy

The mandibular symphysis is limited laterally by the two mental foramens and superiorly by the roots of the incisors, canines and first bicuspids. It is covered by soft tissues consisting of a periosteal layer, mentalis muscle, submucosa and non-keratinised mucosa.

The incisal branches of the mandibular nerve and artery cross the symphyseal region side to side, giving branches to the anterior teeth. The bone in this region is usually dense.[7]

Previous studies have reported that the average bone volume obtained from a symphyseal harvest is 4.71ml, and the average size of cortico-cancellous block measures 20.9x9.9x6.9mm.[18]

Surgical Procedure

Anaesthesia

Harvesting of chin grafts is usually done under local anaesthesia,[19] although intravenous sedation can be used in selected cases.

Local infiltration and blocking of both mental nerves should be done to reduce intraoperative bleeding.

Access

There are two different approaches to gain access to the symphyseal region (Fig 3-1). The sulcular incision is achieved by following the

junction of the keratinised mucosa with the anterior teeth. The incision is made with a No 11 or No 15 blade, separating the papillae with care (Fig 3-2 a, b). Magnification is strongly recommended to avoid tears. Two relieving incisions are made at the level of the canines or first bicuspids (Fig 3-3 a, b).

The vestibular incision is created 5mm below the keratinised mucosa limit to allow further suturing. Mucosa, muscle and periosteum are cut in a through-and-through fashion (Fig 3-4 a, b).

Although the sulcular incision is time-consuming, postoperative oedema and pain are significantly reduced due to maintenance of periosteal and muscle integrity. The only contraindication for the sulcular approach is severe periodontal disease.

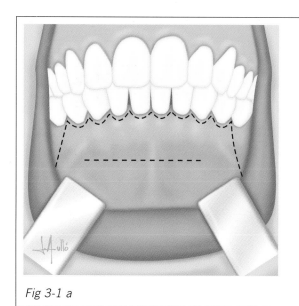
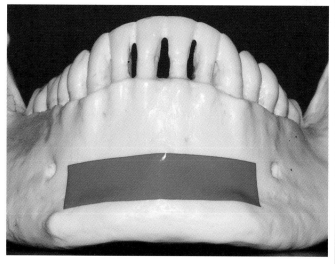

Fig 3-1 a *Fig 3-1 b*

Fig 3-1 (a, b) Sulcular and vestibular incisions allow access to the chin area.

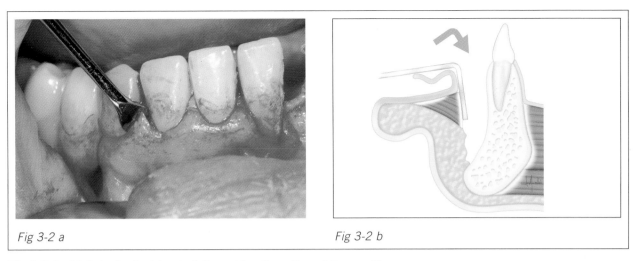

Fig 3-2 a

Fig 3-2 b

Fig 3-2 (a, b) Sulcular incision is followed by dissection of the papillae.

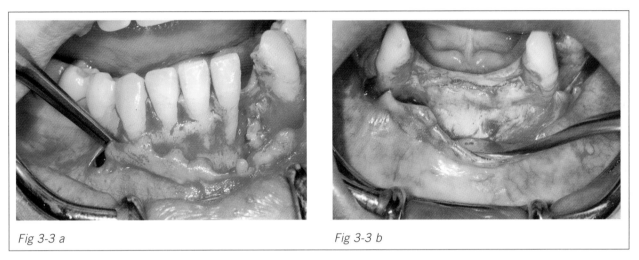

Fig 3-3 a

Fig 3-3 b

Fig 3-3 (a, b) Two cases showing approach to the area. Papillae must be preserved. Relieving incisions should avoid the expected exit of the mental nerve.

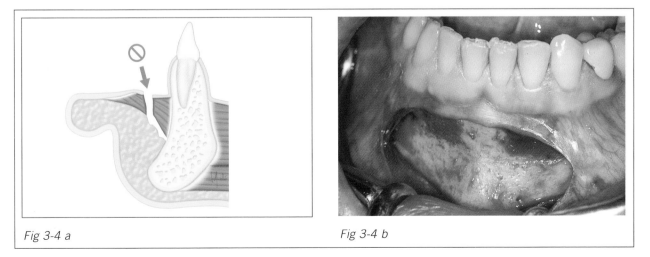

Fig 3-4 a

Fig 3-4 b

Fig 3-4 (a, b) Vestibular incisions are faster but cause more morbidity and impair postoperative recovery.

In both cases subperiosteal dissection is made with care, preserving the integrity of papillae and periosteum. When approaching the inferior border, muscular insertions appear and a sharp periosteal elevator is strongly recommended to detach them from the bone. Lateral subperiosteal dissection proceeds until reaching the exit of the mental nerve on both sides. Preserving dissection under the periosteal layer avoids injury to the nerve.

Harvesting Procedure

To proceed safely to the donor area the '5s' rule should be followed, staying 5mm away from root apices, mental foramen and inferior border of the mandible respectively (Fig 3-5 a, b).

Different methods of graft procurement can be used, depending on the required amount of bone and the size of the defect.

When corticocancellous blocks are needed, careful analysis of the recipient or defective area is required to match the amount of bone grafted to the actual needs.

The choice of instruments at this stage is as follows:

- Fissure bur (No. 702 - a cheap but very effective instrument. Provides very sensitive control of the cut and makes a wide enough groove to allow further positioning of the chisel (Fig 3-6 a, b).

- Saw-preferably an oscillating one. Makes thin cuts that should be convergent (extrusive) (Fig 3-7 a, b).

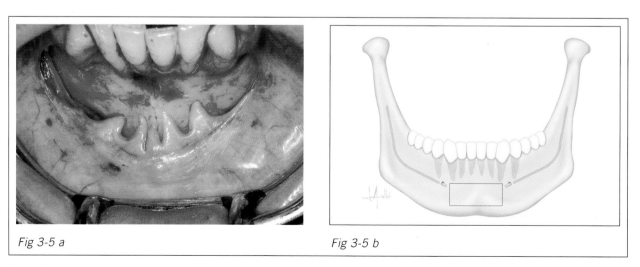

Fig 3-5 a

Fig 3-5 b

Fig 3-5 (a, b) The '5s' rule, staying 5mm away from the apex, the nerves, and the base.

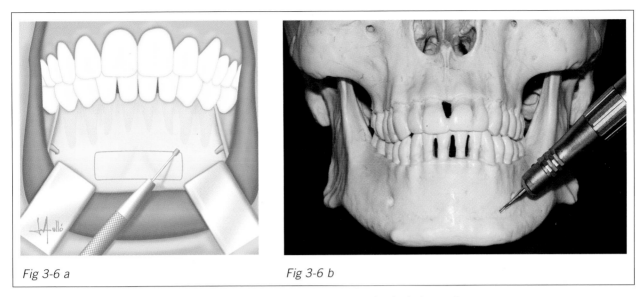

Fig 3-6 a

Fig 3-6 b

Fig 3-6 (a, b) Fissure bur and hand piece are very effective in 'designing' the graft.

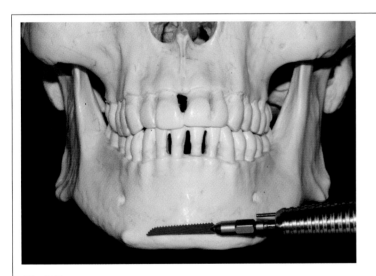

Fig 3-7 a

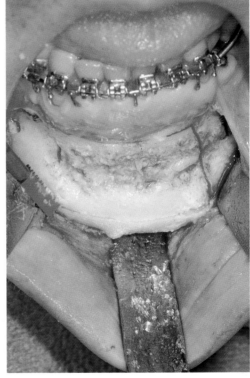

Fig 3-7 (a, b) Saw and blades allow thin cuts with minimal trauma.

Fig 3-7 b

- Disc - acts as a saw, making very thin cuts. It is essential to have a guard to protect soft tissues. Even when protected it is a quite dangerous instrument and, unless tightly controlled, chances of damaging surrounding tissues are high (Fig 3-8 a-c).

- Trephines - indicated when small cores of corticocancellous bone are needed. Depending on the trephine diameter, cores may range between 4-10mm (Fig 3-9 a-e).

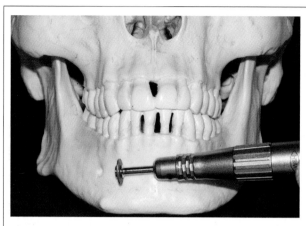

Fig 3-8 a

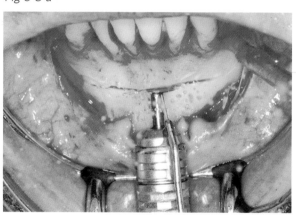

Fig 3-8 b

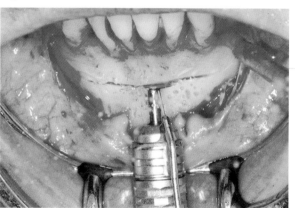

Fig 3-8 (a-c) Disc and handpiece are also very effective but should be used with care to avoid running into soft tissues.

Fig 3-8 c

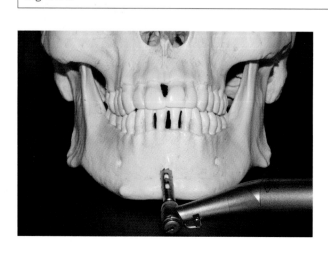

Fig 3-9 (a) Trephines of different diameter are indicated when small cores of bone are needed (for instance, to fill cavities).

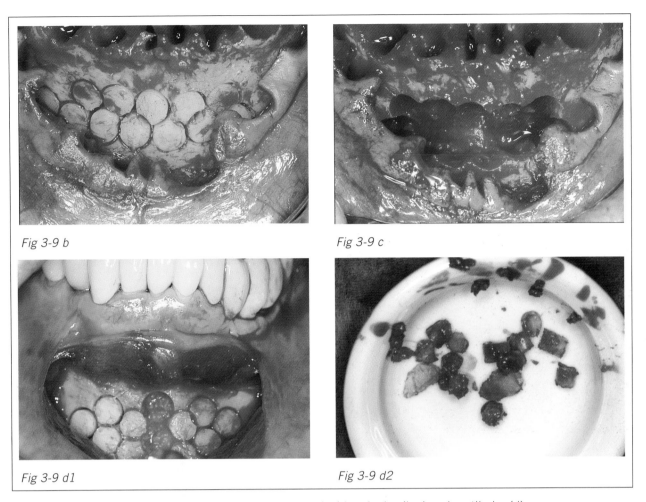

Fig 3-9 b

Fig 3-9 c

Fig 3-9 d1

Fig 3-9 d2

Fig 3-9 (b-d) Two cases of trephine harvest are illustrated with sulcular (b,c) and vestibular (d) access.

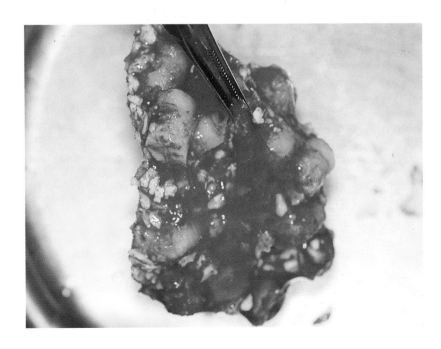

Fig 3-9 (e) Bone cores may be mixed with PRP for easy management.

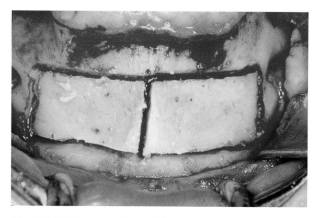

Fig 3-10 Total symphyseal harvesting is facilitated by cutting the graft in the middle reducing the risk of graft fracture.

In most cases the desired block will be a corticocancellous one, thus leaving the lingual cortex intact. This approach limits the available bone but avoids violation of the floor of the mouth with its inherent vascular risks.

Irrespective of the instrument used to design the osteotomy, it is not difficult to feel the inner cortical limit. In our experience, fissure burs give adequate control of the cut.

When maximum harvesting from the area is desired it is useful to create a midline vertical osteotomy to facilitate elevation of the graft (Fig 3-10).[18]

Once the osteotomy has been designed, a sharp curved osteotome should be inserted in the crease and carefully bent to allow dislodgement of the block (Fig 3-11 a, b).

After harvesting of the block any remaining cancellous bone can be removed with bone curettes.

Before trimming and fixing the graft, we strongly recommend closing the donor area in order to avoid excessive bleeding and reduce the risk of infection. Moderate bleeding can be anticipated at this site but usually ceases by compression

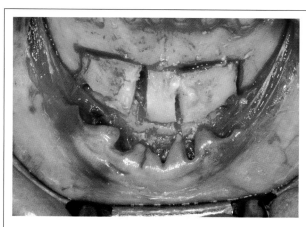

Fig 3-11 a

Fig 3-11 (a, b) Introducing and bending a chisel in the previously made grooves aids in freeing the graft.

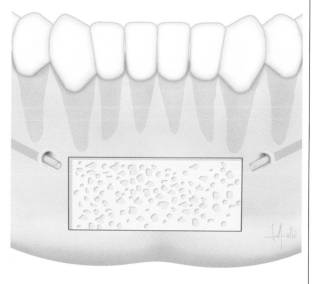

Fig 3-11 b

with gauze within a few minutes. Should it persist, different haemostatic agents or a collagen membrane can be used. For this purpose, during the past few years we have been using PRP with good and fast results.

In elderly people we mix PRP with bovine inorganic matrix to favour regeneration at this level (Fig 3-12 a, b). In younger patients we only place the plasma to aid in haemostasis but leave the future regeneration of the site to the periosteum from the flap.

When a vestibular approach is employed, suturing is completed with a 4/0 resorbable run-

ning suture or a 5/0 interrupted suture to close the wound in the case of a sulcular incision (Fig 3-13 a-c).

Once removed, the bone graft has to be trimmed and perfectly adapted to the recipient area. This is especially important in membranous bone blocks due to the rigidity of the bone. If adaptation is defective, empty spaces will remain between the graft and the recipient site, facilitating ingrowth of fibrous tissue or, worse, infection. These grafts can be easily carved to intimately adapt to defects.[18]

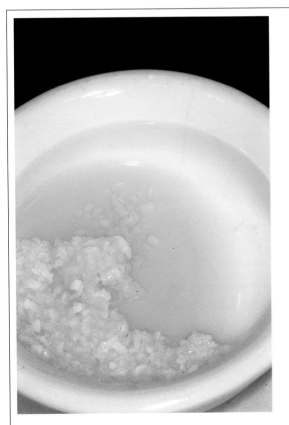

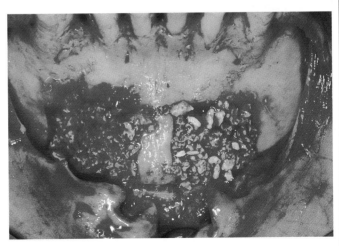

Fig 3-12 (a, b) Filling the donor site with bovine bone matrix and PRP may accelerate regeneration in the area.

Fig 3-12 a   *Fig 3-12 b*

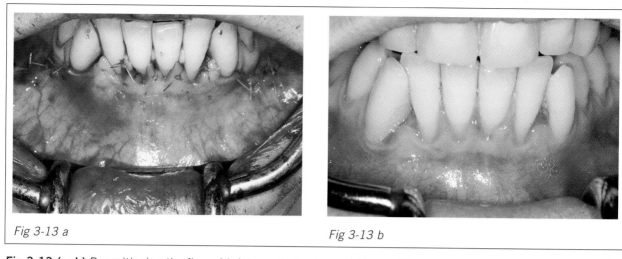

Fig 3-13 a

Fig 3-13 b

Fig 3-13 (a, b) Repositioning the flap with interrupted sutures at the papillae.

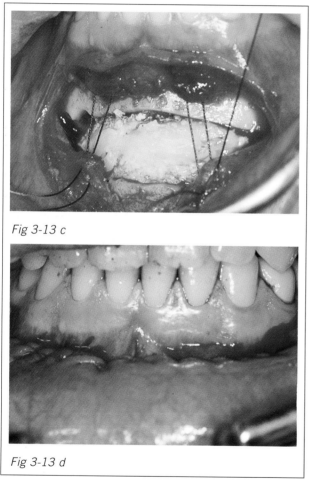

Fig 3-13 c

Fig 3-13 d

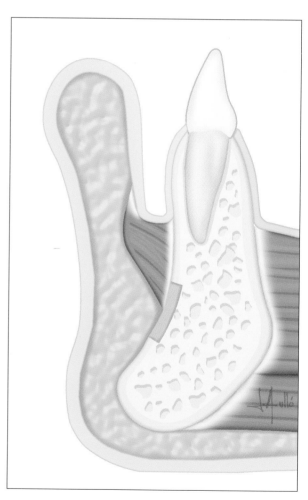

Fig 3-13 (c, d) Muscles have to be sutured together in a separate plane with interrupted sutures before closing the mucosa.

Fig 3-13 (e) The donor site is covered by the composite flap (mucosa-muscle-periosteum).

One compression screw for each block will maintain adequate fixation at the recipient site (Fig 3-14 a-c). Grafts have to be trimmed and adapted to fit perfectly in the defects (Fig 3-15 a, b).

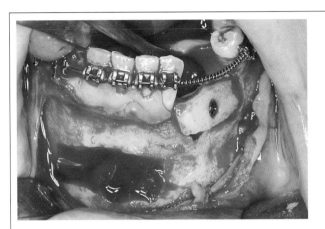

Fig 3-14 a

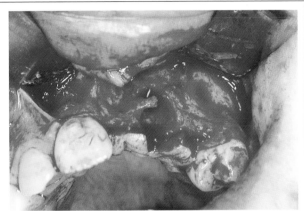

Fig 3-14 b

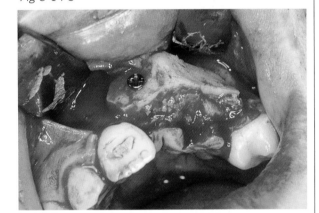

Fig 3-14 (a-c) In most instances a single screw suffices to fix a block.

Fig 3-14 c

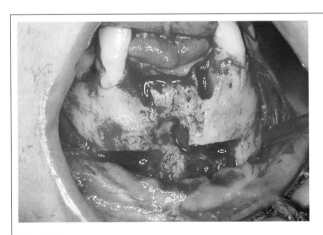

Fig 3-15 a

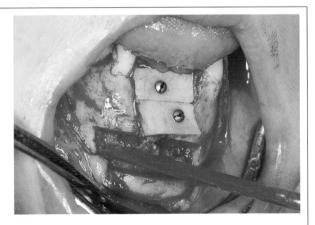

Fig 3-15 b

Fig 3-15 (a, b) Block divided in two and adapted to a crestal defect in the vicinity.

In instances where particulated bone is needed the harvested blocks have to be ground with a bone mill. In these cases we strongly recommend the use of PRP, as its adherent and viscous properties facilitate transportation and adaptation of the graft (Fig 3-16).

As previously mentioned, the waiting period between graft fixation and insertion of fixtures varies between 0 and 6 months.

Immediate insertion of fixtures can be undertaken when the reconstruction is judged to provide enough stability for them (Fig 3-17 a-l). If fixture insertion is delayed, two to three months will suffice in cases in which blocks have been used and four to six months in cases of particulated grafts. In the last two instances fixation screws will be removed at implant placement (Fig 3-18 a-m).

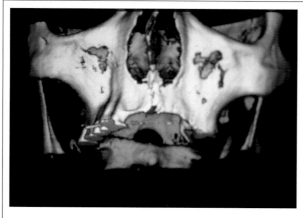

Fig 3-16 Trephined bone from the chin mixed with PRP.

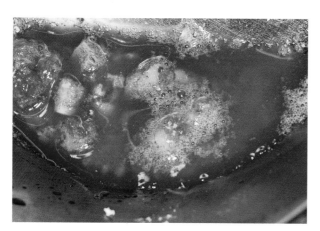

Fig 3-17 a

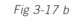

Fig 3-17 b

Fig 3-17 (a, b) Simultaneous graft placement and implant insertion can be done if reconstruction is stable enough. This case shows a severe AP atrophy (Cawood class IV) of the anterior maxilla.

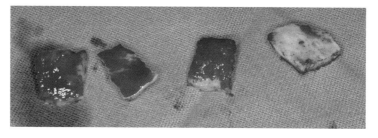

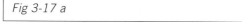

Fig 3-17 (c) Four blocks were harvested from the chin.

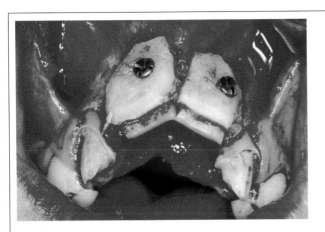

Fig 3-17 d

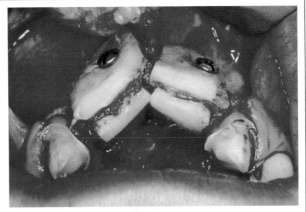

Fig 3-17 e

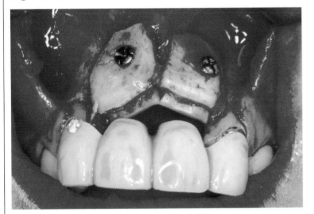

Fig 3-17 f

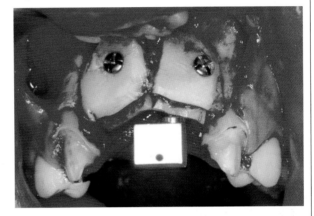

Fig 3-17 g

Fig 3-17 (d-h) Two blocks on each side of the atrophic ridge were secured with tri-cortical screws. Integrity of the reconstruction warrants immediate fixture insertion following the surgical guide. This is feasible when fixation screws do not interfere with implant direction.

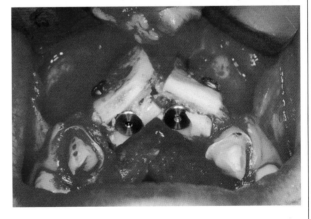

Fig 3-17 h

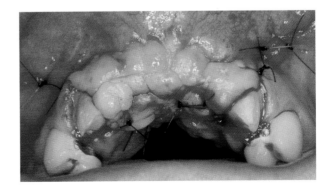

Fig 3-17 (i) Primary closure with interrupted sutures.

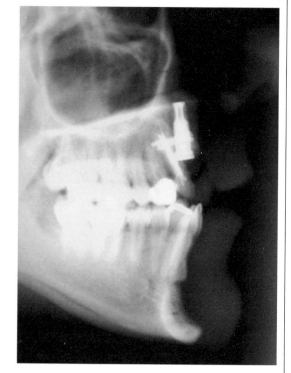

Fig 3-17 j

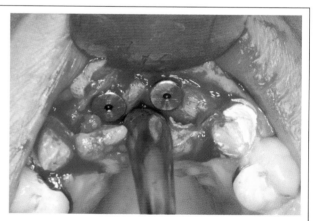

Fig 3-17 (j, k) Radiographs showing adequate position and inclination of the fixtures.

Fig 3-17 k

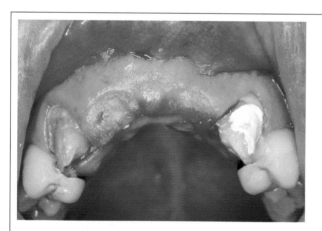

Fig 3-17 l

Fig 3-17 m

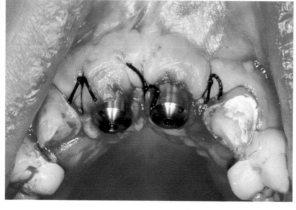

Fig 3-17 n

Fig 3-17 (l-n) Re-entry and abutment connection.

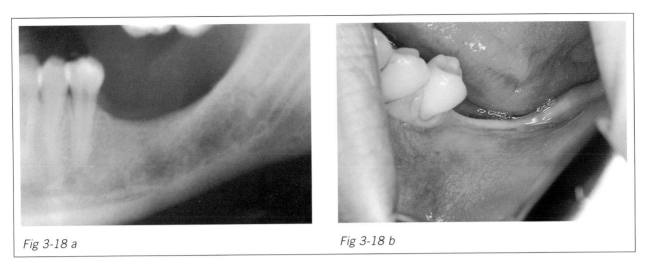

Fig 3-18 a

Fig 3-18 b

Fig 3-18 (a, b) Edentulous segment in the mandible with vertical atrophy.

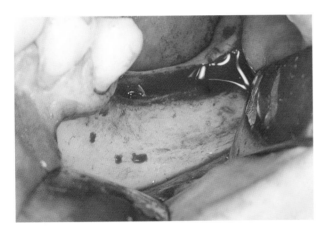

Fig 3-18 (c) Crestal incision mesially relieved is followed by careful subperiosteal dissection.

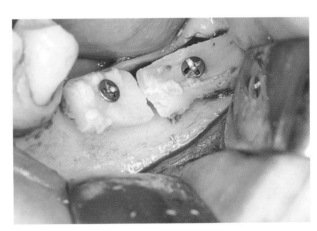

Fig 3-18 (d) Two blocks from the chin secured with screws improving the verical defect.

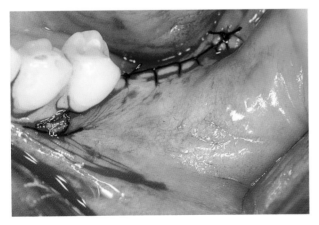

Fig 3-18 (e) Watertight closure with running sutures.

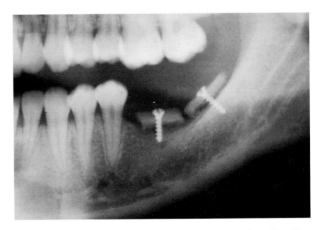

Fig 3-18 (f) Panoramic X-ray taken two weeks after the procedure.

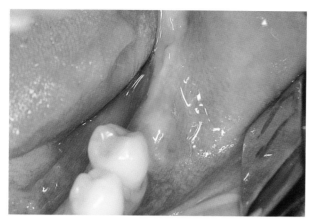

Fig 3-18 (g) Clinical aspect three months after the procedure.

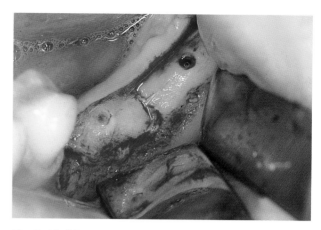

Fig 3-18 (h) Grafts are well integrated at the host site, allowing screw removal.

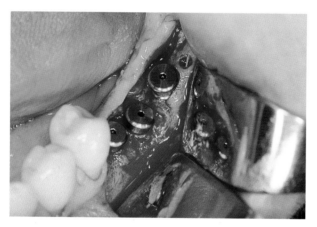

Fig 3-18 (i) Three 10mm fixtures are placed.

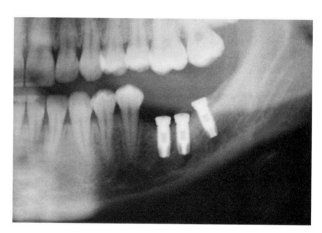

Fig 3-18 (j) Control panoramic X-ray. Nowadays we would leave the fixtures connected with the healing caps at this point.

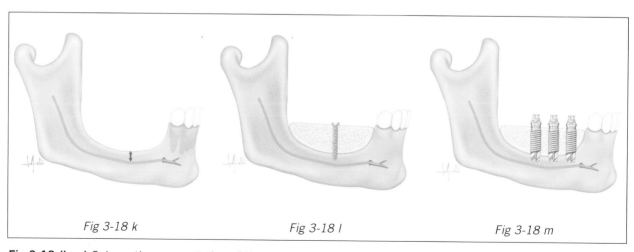

Fig 3-18 k   *Fig 3-18 l*   *Fig 3-18 m*

Fig 3-18 (k-m) Schematic representation of the procedure.

Postoperative Care

Extraoral compression and cryotherapy of the area is strongly recommended to avoid excessive swelling. Antibiotic as well as anti-inflammatory drugs are prescribed as well as a soft toothbrush to clean the surgical area.

Complications

Intraoperatory

Neural: Careful identification of both of the mental nerves will allow protection and avoid them being compressed or stretched. The assisting surgeon or nurse will in most instances be responsible for separation of the flap and preservation of nerve integrity, especially during the osteotomies.

The incisal branch of the mandibular nerve runs transversely deep in the symphysis and will be exposed when deep harvesting of cancellous bone is undertaken in the area. Severing of this branch will produce varying degrees of subjective neural dysfunction.

Dental: There is a potential risk for damaging mandibular tooth roots or the mental nerve. Careful radiographic examination with panoramic X-ray and possibly CT scan will prevent most of these complications. Leaving 5mm of security distance between the apex of the canines and the upper osteotomy is mandatory.

Postoperatory

Swelling: Variable degrees of swelling can be anticipated when harvesting bone from the symphyseal region. When an intrasulcular incision and subperiosteal dissection are employed, avoiding transection of muscle fibres from the chin region, less swelling and pain can be anticipated.

Clinical Applications

Chin grafts may be useful in the management of different reconstructive procedures both in the maxilla and mandible (Fig 3-19 to 3-31).

We prefer this donor site in cases where small to medium-sized blocks are needed.

The main indications for these grafts are inlay/onlay grafting at the anterior maxilla,[19,20,21] inlay/onlay grafting at the posterior maxilla and onlay vestibular/crestal grafting in the mandible.

43

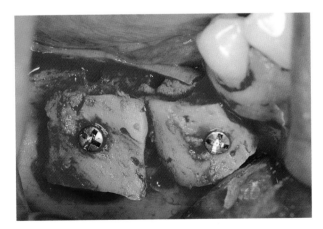

Fig 3-19 (a) Vestibular defect at the posterior mandible, managed with two onlay grafts from the chin.

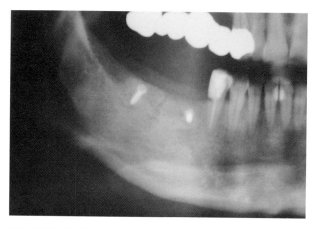

Fig 3-19 (b) Panoramic X-ray.

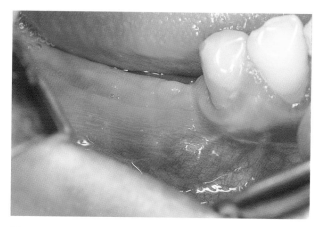

Fig 3-19 (c) Clinical aspect three months later.

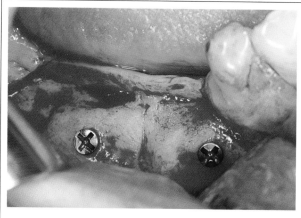

Fig 3-19 d

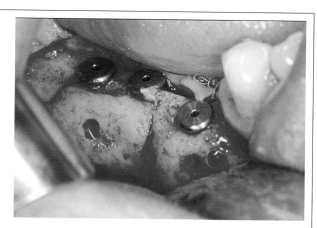

Fig 3-19 e

Fig 3-19 (d, e) Screw removal and fixture placement.

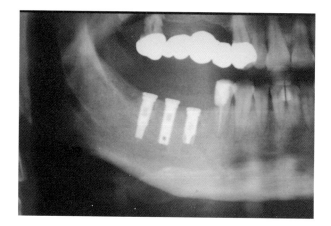

Fig 3-19 (f) Control panoramic X-ray.

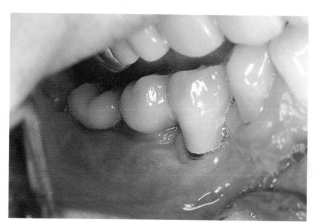

Fig 3-19 (g) Final result.

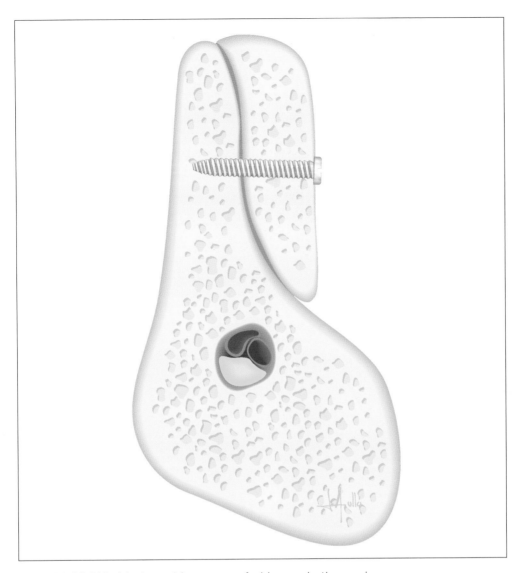

Fig 3-19 (h) Chin block used in a veneer fashion, as in the previous case.

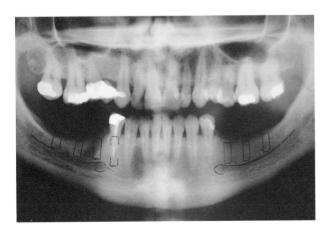

Fig 3-20 (a) Bilaterally edentulous mandible with vertical defects.

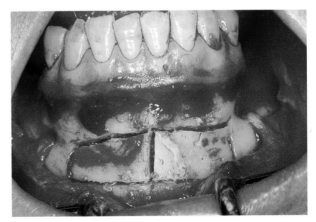

Fig 3-20 (b) Vestibular incision in continuity with the bilateral crestal incisions gives access to the symphyseal region, and allows design of the grafts needed. Note the exit of both mental nerves.

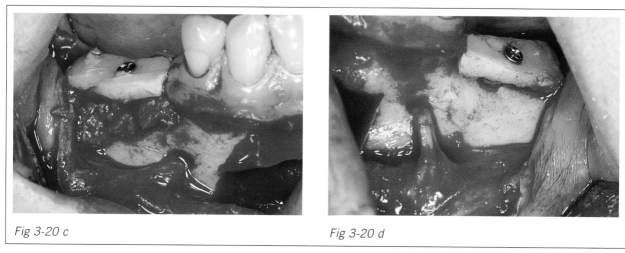

Fig 3-20 c

Fig 3-20 d

Fig 3-20 (c, d) Graft fixation on both sides. Extra cancellous bone can be harvested from the same site to obliterate empty spaces under the grafts.

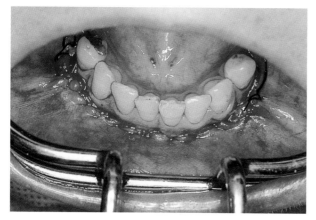

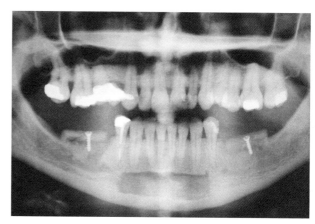

Fig 3-20 (e) Closure of the incisions with running sutures.

Fig 3-20 (f) Control panoramic X-ray showing both the vertically reconstructed areas and the donor site. The '5s' rule can be followed in this image.

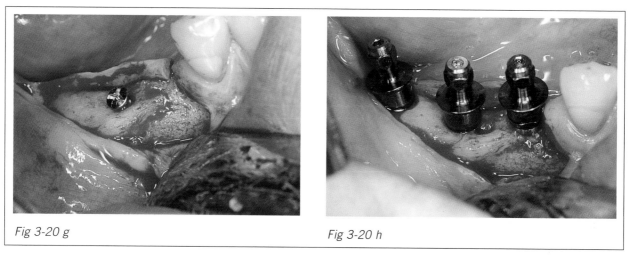

Fig 3-20 g

Fig 3-20 h

Fig 3-20 (g, h) Re-entry three months later showing consolidation of the graft and fixture placement.

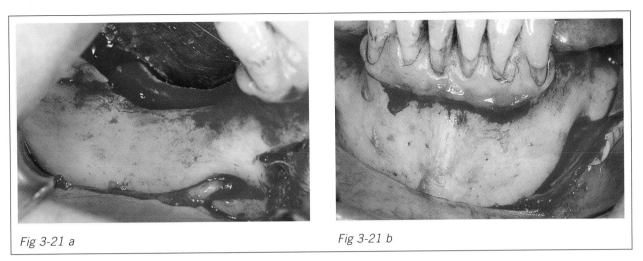

Fig 3-21 a

Fig 3-21 b

Fig 3-21 (a, b) Similar clinical situation with side-to-side approach.

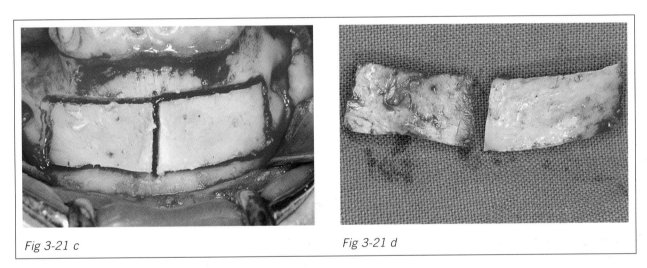

Fig 3-21 c

Fig 3-21 d

Fig 3-21 (c, d) Harvest of two blocks using most of the chin area.

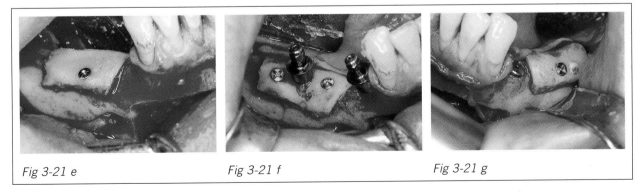

Fig 3-21 e

Fig 3-21 f

Fig 3-21 g

Fig 3-21 (e-g) Fixation of the grafts on both sides. We tried to place an immediate fixture on the right side, provoking a fracture of the graft. Two screws were needed to re-secure it.

Fig 3-21 h

Fig 3-21 i

Fig 3-21 (h,i) Closure.

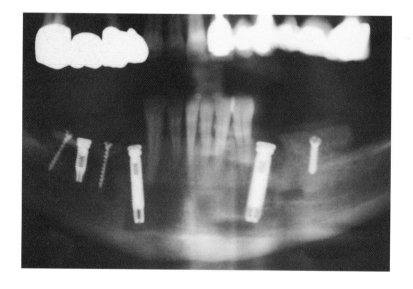

Fig 3-21 (j) Control panoramic X-ray.

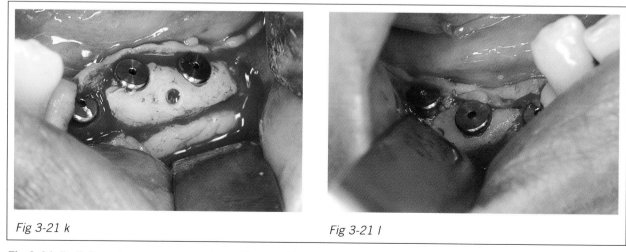

Fig 3-21 k

Fig 3-21 l

Fig 3-21 (k, l) Re-entry, screw removal and fixture placement.

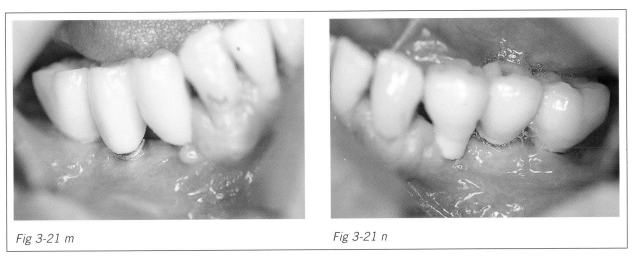

Fig 3-21 m   Fig 3-21 n

Fig 3-21 (m, n) Final restoration.

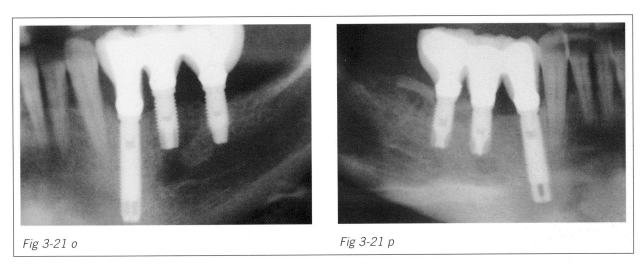

Fig 3-21 o   Fig 3-21 p

Fig 3-21 (o, p) Control radiograph.

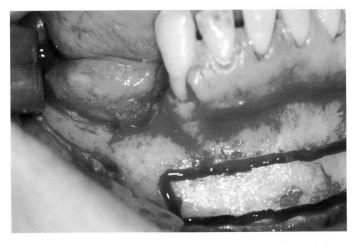

Fig 3-22 (a) Vertical defect at the posterior mandible. A long strip of cortical bone is harvested. Note that the width of the graft is enough to allow future placement of fixtures.

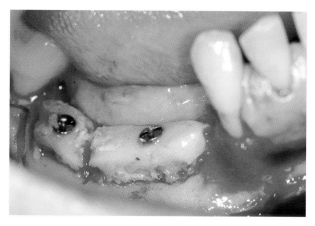

Fig 3-22 (b) The block is divided and adapted to the defect. Two screws are used for fixation with care to avoid invasion of the neurovascular bundle.

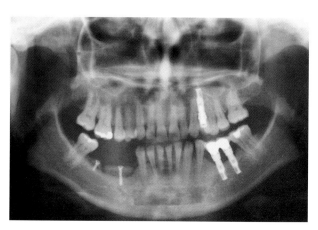

Fig 3-22 (c) Panoramic X-ray showing reconstruction.

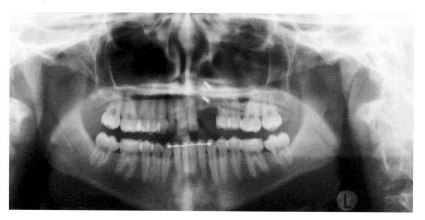

Fig 3-23 (a) This young patient was involved in a traffic accident resulting in avulsion of teeth 22 and 23 and loss of the vestibular alveolar wall at this level. Reconstruction was carried out as an emergency procedure one hour after the accident. The control panoramic X-ray one day after surgery shows screws holding two pieces of bone harvested from the chin.

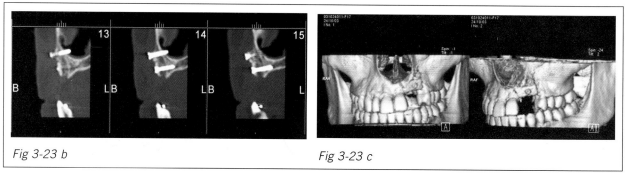

Fig 3-23 b

Fig 3-23 c

Fig 3-23 (b, c) CT scan illustrates both veneer blocks improving transverse dimensions of the crest.

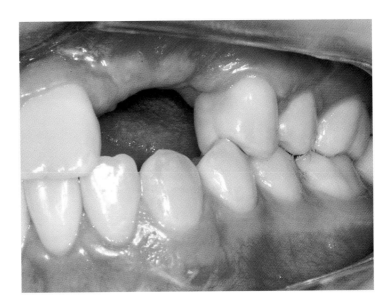

Fig 3-23 (d) Clinical aspect at the time of re-entry.

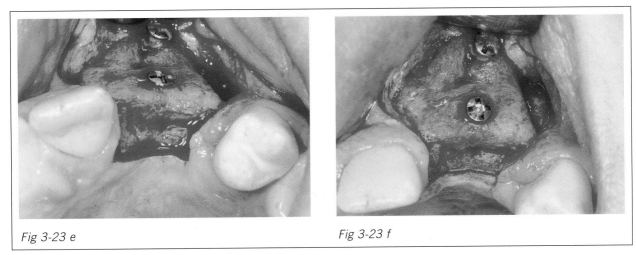

Fig 3-23 e *Fig 3-23 f*

Fig 3-23 (e, f) A full-thickness flap respecting the papillae is designed to favour transport of keratinised mucosa to the buccal side. Note how grafts have been incorporated to the recipient site.

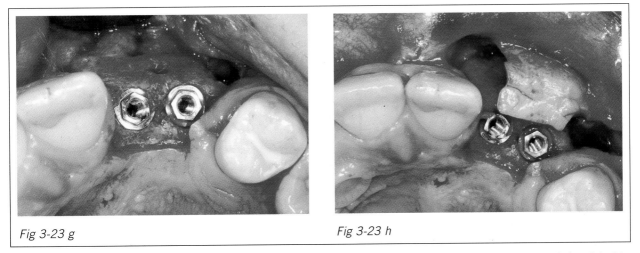

Fig 3-23 g *Fig 3-23 h*

Fig 3-23 (g, h) Two fixtures are placed according to the surgical guide following removal of the screws. It is advisable to maintain the screws until the fixtures have been positioned. This, however, is not possible when the screws are in the way of implant insertion, which was the case in our patient.

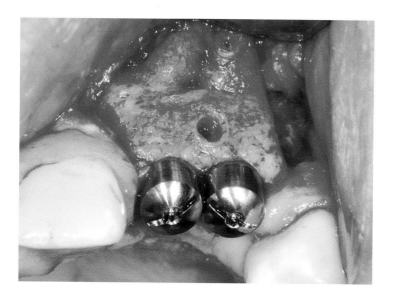

Fig 3-23 (i) Abutment connection is done at this point.

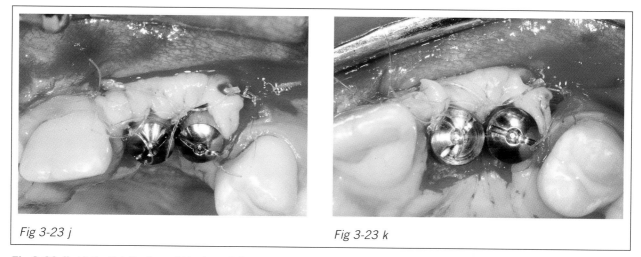

Fig 3-23 j

Fig 3-23 k

Fig 3-23 (j, k) Redistribution of the keratinised mucosa with 'mini-flaps' is done at the vestibular side. This will improve soft tissue volume and architecture.

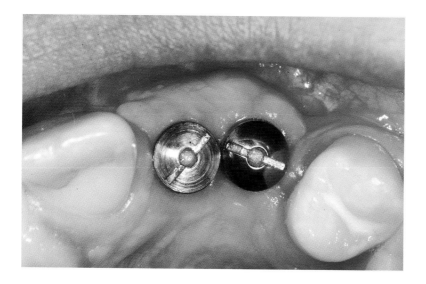

Fig 3-23 (l) Healing after two weeks. Note the improved volume at the buccal side due to bone grafting and soft-tissue management.

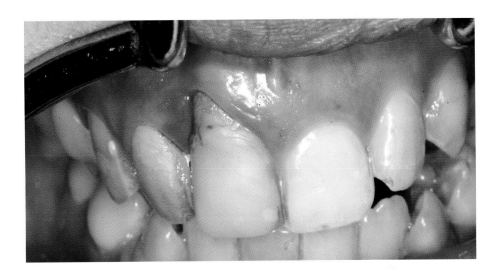

Fig 3-24 (a) Preoperative view of a chronically inflamed tissues and periodontally compromised central incisor.

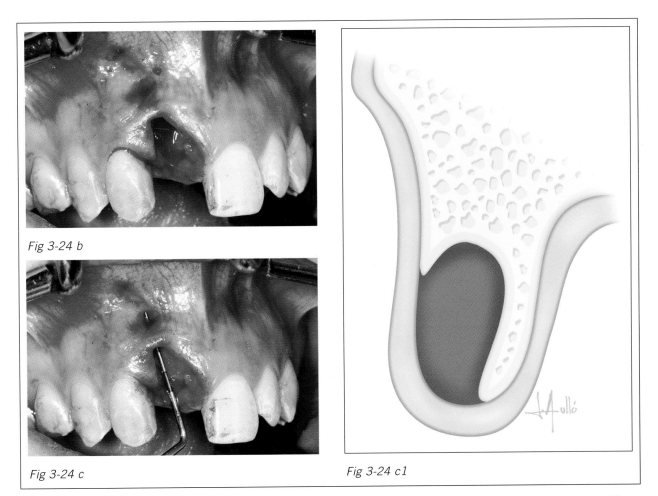

Fig 3-24 b

Fig 3-24 c

Fig 3-24 c1

Fig 3-24 (b, c, c1) Defective soft and hard tissues after tooth removal. A periodontal probe shows absence of buccal bone and presence of a fistula.

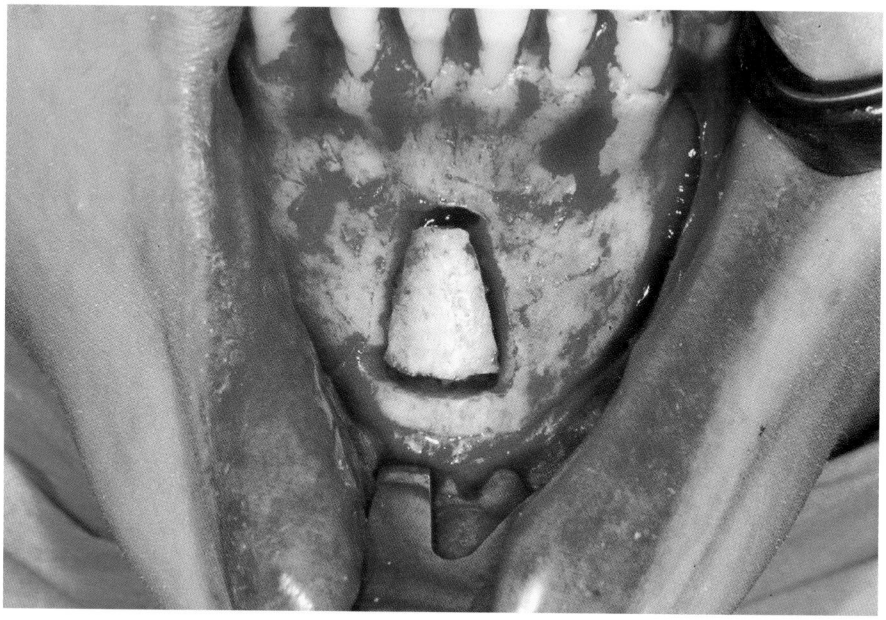

Fig 3-24 d

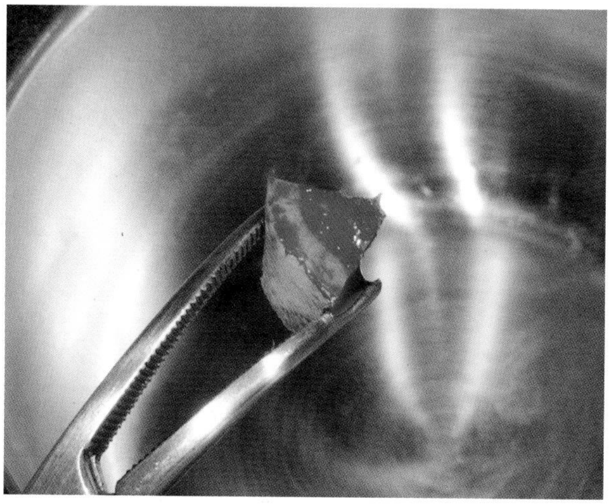

Fig 3-24 e

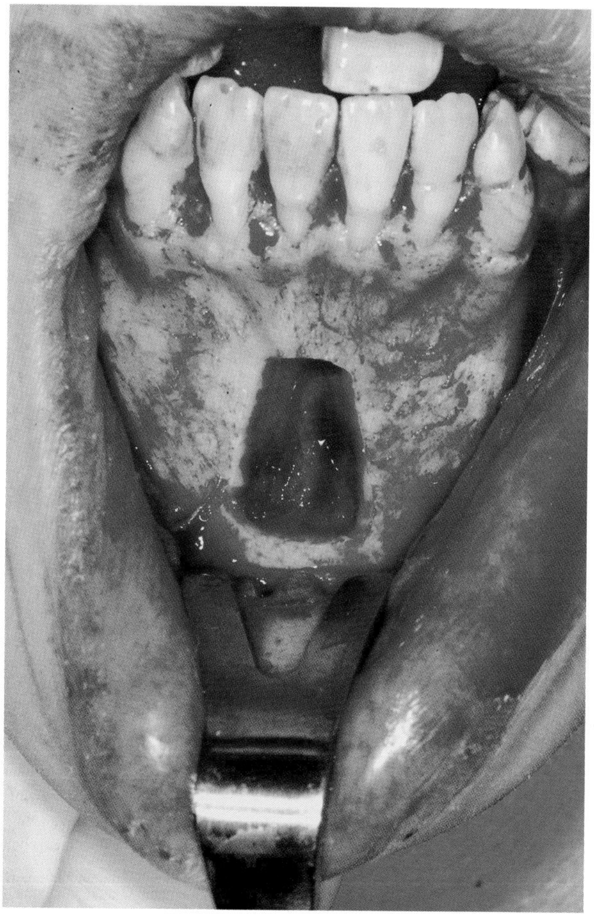

Fig 3-24 f

Fig 3-24 (d-f) A symphyseal bone graft is harvested. Note how the shape of the block fits that of the defect tridimensionally.

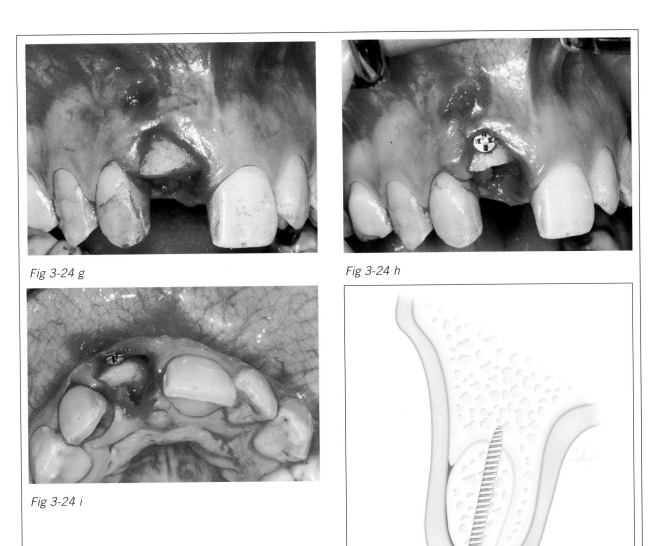

Fig 3-24 g

Fig 3-24 h

Fig 3-24 i

Fig 3-24 i1

Fig 3-24 (g-i1) The block is impacted in the residual alveolus with the cortical aspect facing buccally. A screw aids in graft stabilisation.

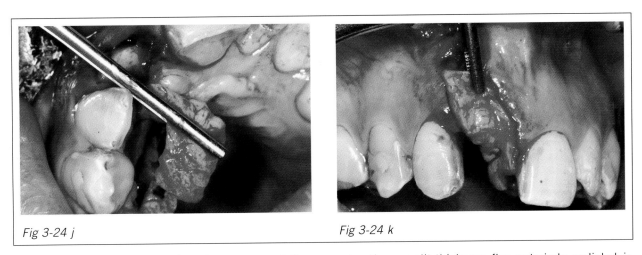

Fig 3-24 j

Fig 3-24 k

Fig 3-24 (j, k) To achieve adequate coverage of the reconstruction a split-thickness flap anteriorly pedicled is designed and rotated buccally to cover the graft.

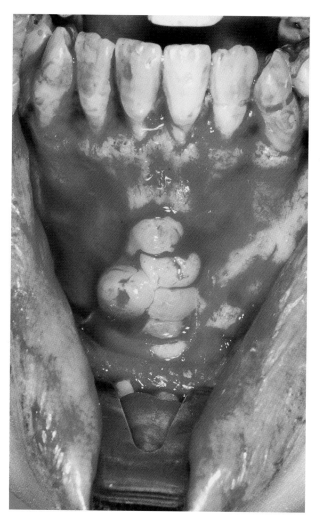

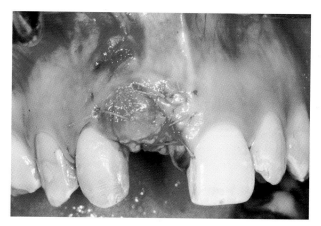

Fig 3-24 (m) The flap is secured in place with 5/0 resorbable sutures. Note how the distal end of the flap is sutured apically to cover the old fistula.

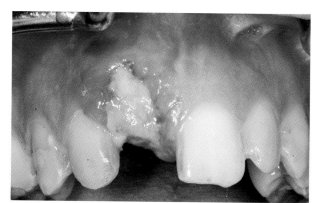

Fig 3-24 (l) The donor site is filled up with PRP to enhance healing and minimise bruising.

Fig 3-24 (n) One week postoperatively the submucosal flap is in the process of mucous metaplasia.

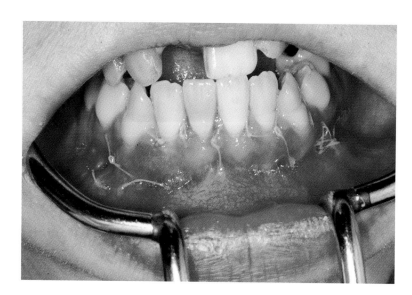

Fig 3-24 (o) Donor site.

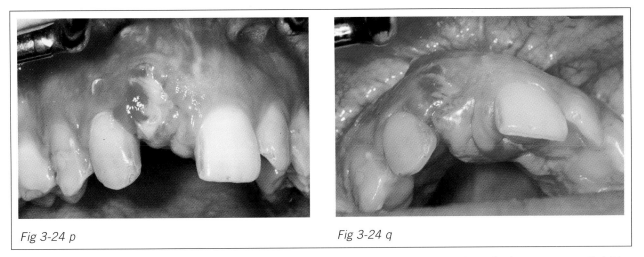

Fig 3-24 p

Fig 3-24 q

Fig 3-24 (p, q) Three weeks after the procedure metaplasia of the flap is completed. There is, however, a small dehiscence over the screw.

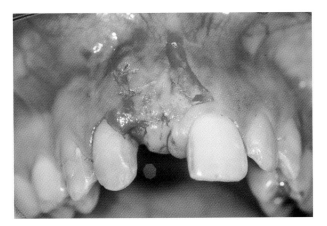

Fig 3-24 (r) A partial thickness mucosal flap pedicled apically suffices to cover the dehiscence.

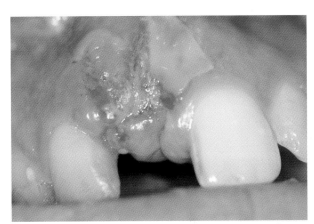

Fig 3-24 (s) One week postoperatively.

Fig 3-24 (t) Three weeks postoperatively. Compared with initial pictures, crestal height and width have been reconstructed with adequate soft-tissue coverage.

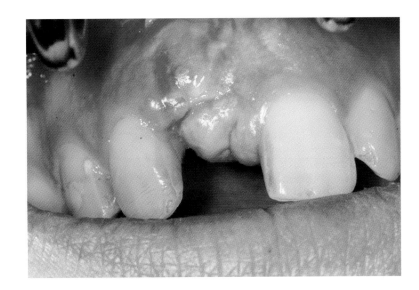

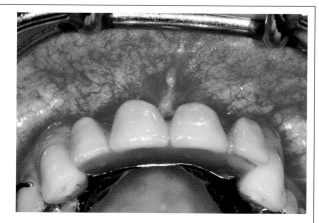

Fig 3-25 a

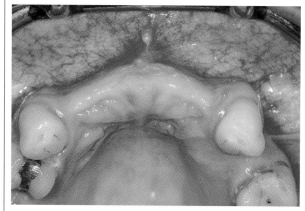

Fig 3-25 b

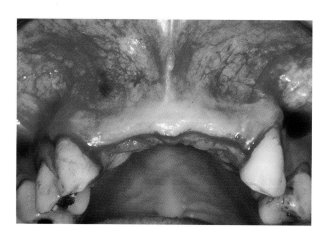

Fig 3-25 c

Fig 3-25 (a-c) Absence of four incisors. The partially removable denture has caused severe anteroposterior atrophy of the crest. A crestal split with inlay grafting is programmed.

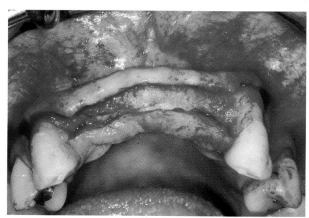

Fig 3-25 (d) A crestal incision.

Fig 3-25 (e) Minimal periosteal stripping warrants adequate blood supply to the vestibular bony flap.

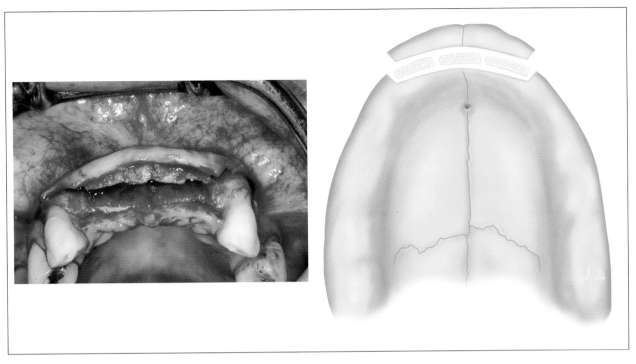

Fig 3-25 (f) A mid-crestal osteotomy is done to allow splitting.

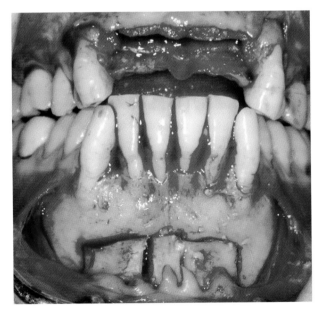

Fig 3-25 (g) Two blocks are harvested from the chin to be used as interpositional grafts.

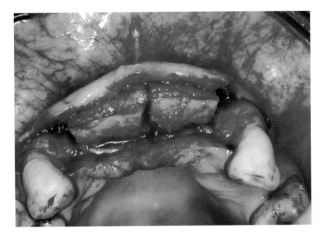

Fig 3-25 (h) Following graft insertion, a normal crestal width is achieved.

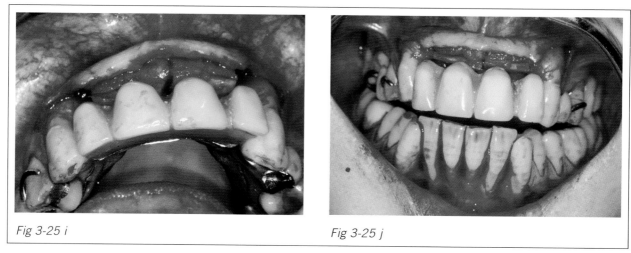

Fig 3-25 i

Fig 3-25 j

Fig 3-25 (i, j) The old partially removable denture in place illustrates the achievement of an adequate crestal anatomy.

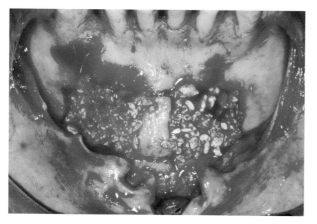

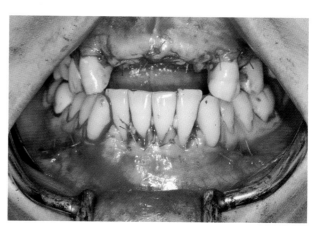

Fig 3-25 (k) The donor site is reconstructed with bovine inorganic bone mixed with PRP.

Fig 3-25 (l) Watertight closure of the flaps without tension.

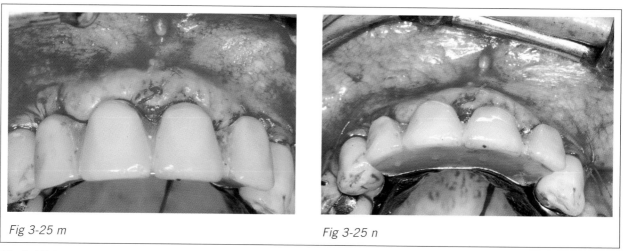

Fig 3-25 m

Fig 3-25 n

Fig 3-25 (m, n) The partial denture has been trimmed and adapted to the new anatomy.

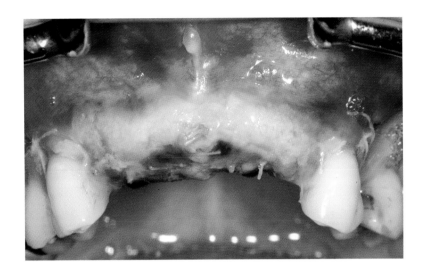

Fig 3-25 (o) Clinical aspect one week postoperatively.

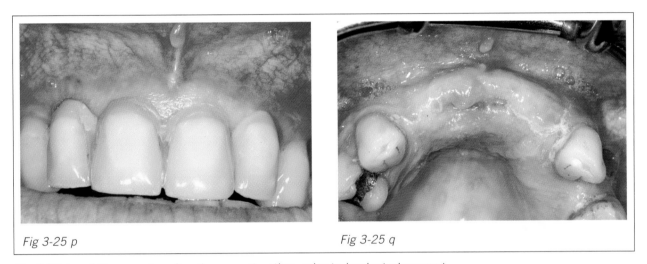

Fig 3-25 p

Fig 3-25 q

Fig 3-25 (p, q) Two months after the reconstruction, prior to implant placement.

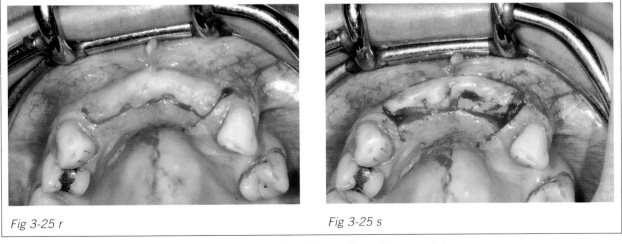

Fig 3-25 r

Fig 3-25 s

Fig 3-25 (r, s) A limited mid-crestal incision respecting the papillae allows crestal access.

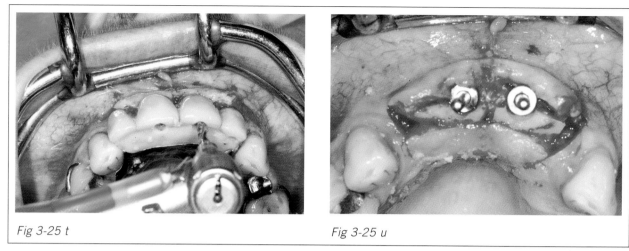

Fig 3-25 t   *Fig 3-25 u*

Fig 3-25 (t, u) Fixtures are placed following a surgical stent.

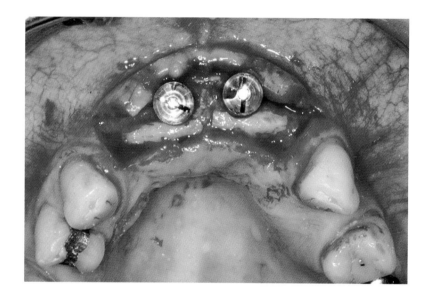

Fig 3-25 (v) Abutment connection.

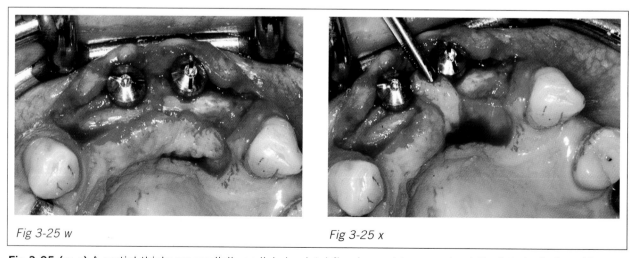

Fig 3-25 w   *Fig 3-25 x*

Fig 3-25 (w, x) A partial thickness medially pedicled palatal flap is used to reconstruct the interincisal papilla.

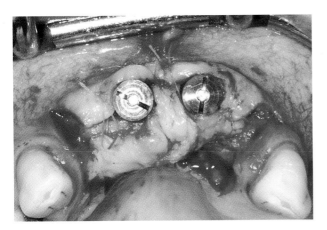

Fig 3-25 (y) Tailoring of the flaps.

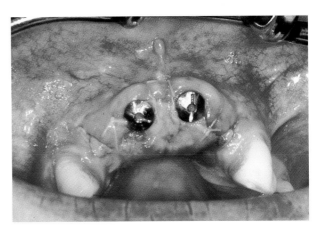

Fig 3-25 (z) One week postoperatively.

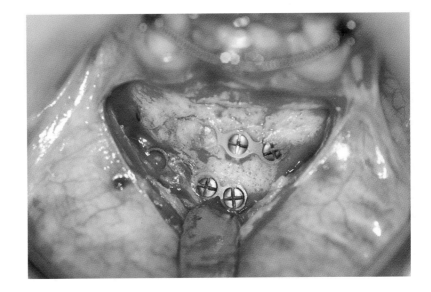

Fig 3-26 (a) Old mandibular fracture treated with rigid fixation. Note how bone in-growth has partially covered the plates and screws. Bone reconstruction has to be completed around the inferior lateral incisors.

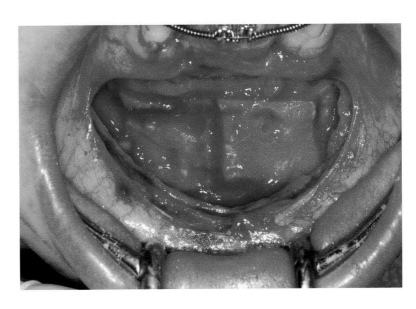

Fig 3-26 (b) After removal of the plates and screws, two blocks are harvested from the same area. Harvesting is done with fissure burs and chisels.

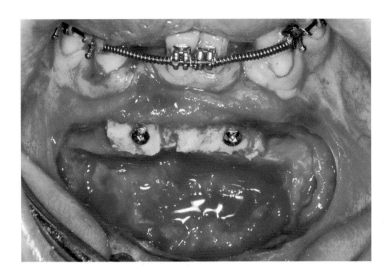

Fig 3-26 (c) Blocks are fixed in position with compression screws.

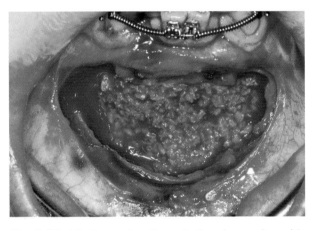

Fig 3-26 (d) Reconstruction at the donor site with bovine anorganic substitute and PRP.

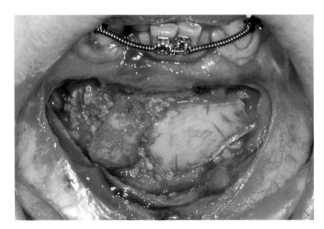

Fig 3-26 (e) A septoplasty was carried out simultaneously. Cartilage grafts from the septum were harvested and used as barrier 'membranes' since the periosteum in this area was severely disrupted due to previous trauma.

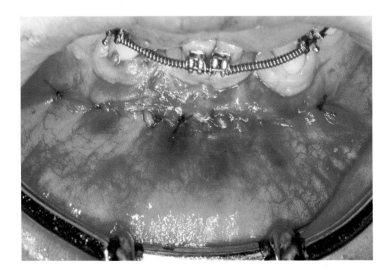

Fig 3-26 (f) Closure.

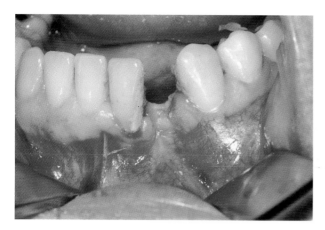

Fig 3-27 (a) 3-wall defect after excision of an odontoma related to a lower-left lateral incisor.

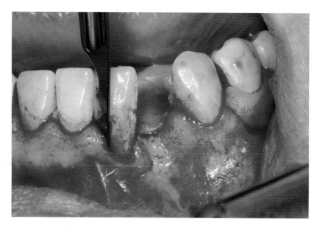

Fig 3-27 (b) Sulcular incision is done with a No. 15c blade with care to preserve the papillae.

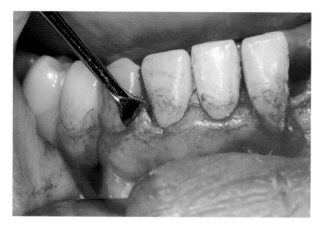

Fig 3-27 (c) A sharp papilla dissector aids in elevating the flap.

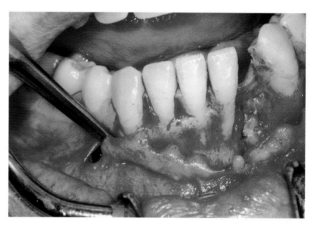

Fig 3-27 (d) Two relieving incisions at the level of the canines allow reflecting the flap without tension.

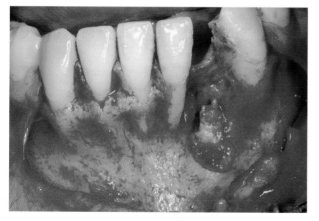

Fig 3-27 (e) The size of the defect with incomplete fibrous healing can be depicted in this image.

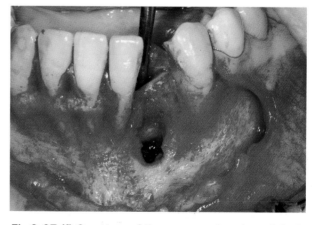

Fig 3-27 (f) Curettage of the area reveals a deep defect.

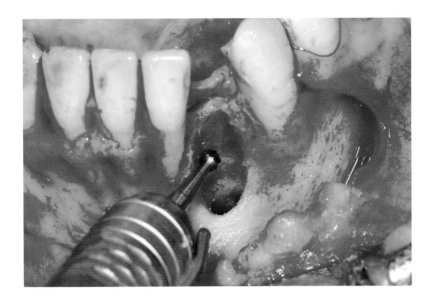

Fig 3-27 (g) A round bur is used to 'activate' the recipient site and eliminate fibrous remnants.

Fig 3-27 (h, x) A triangular bone block is harvested with a fissure bur and a chisel. Extra cancellous bone is harvested through the same window to fill the deep hole at the recipient site. The block is then fixed with a single screw in a compressive fashion to the lingual cortex. Remodelling of sharp edges is done with a round bur. Note how AP and vertical defects have been corrected.

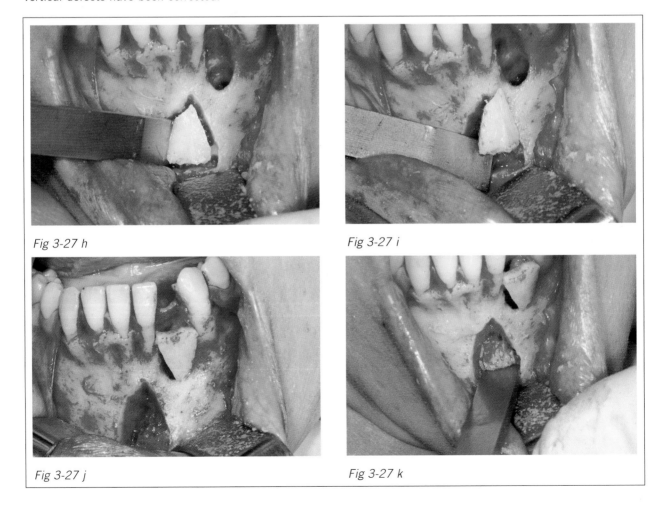

Fig 3-27 h

Fig 3-27 i

Fig 3-27 j

Fig 3-27 k

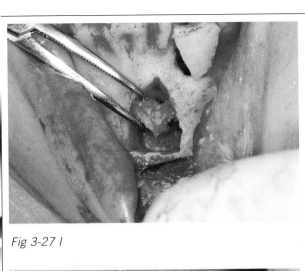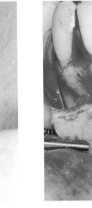

Fig 3-27 l

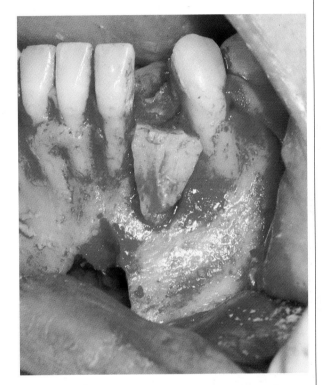

Fig 3-27 m

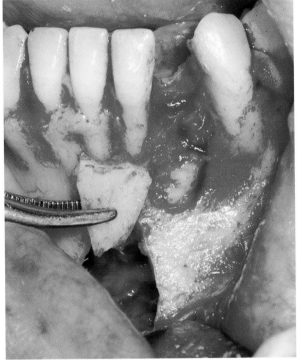

Fig 3-27 n

Fig 3-27 o

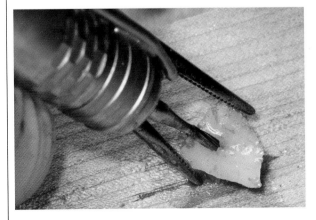

Fig 3-27 p

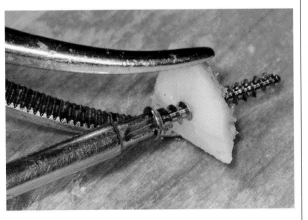

Fig 3-27 q

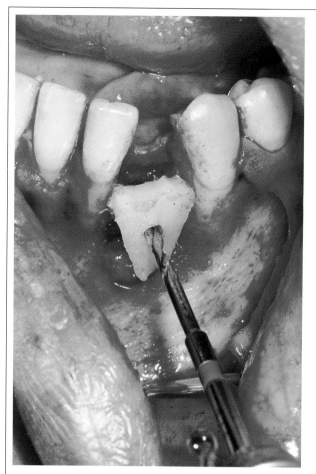

Fig 3-27 r

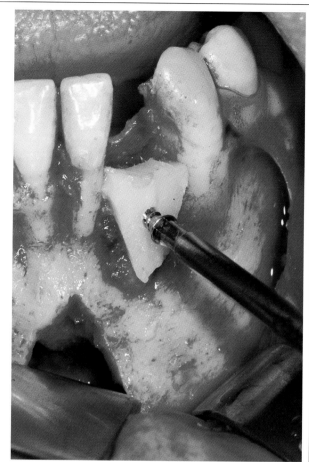

Fig 3-27 s

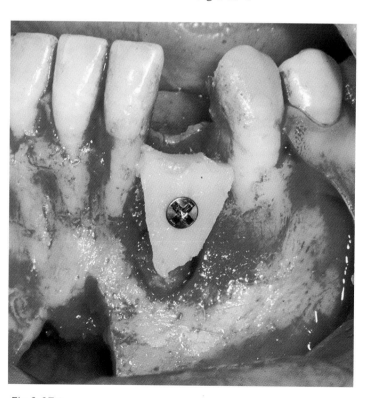

Fig 3-27 t

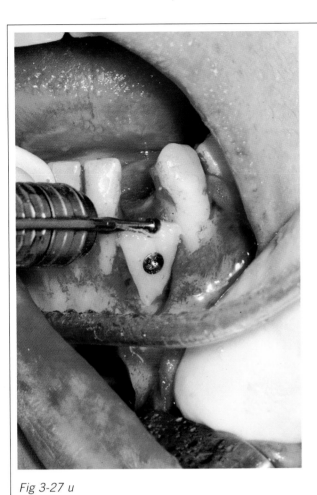

Fig 3-27 u

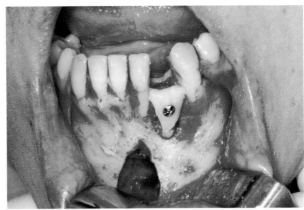

Fig 3-27 v

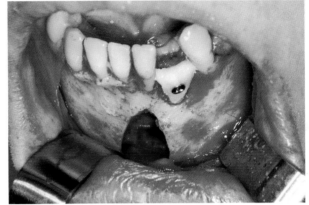

Fig 3-27 x

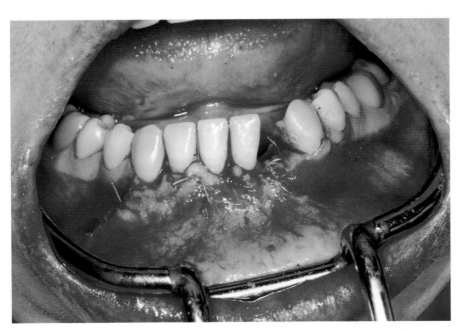

Fig 3-27 (y) It is of utmost importance to achieve soft-tissue coverage and sealing of the reconstructions.

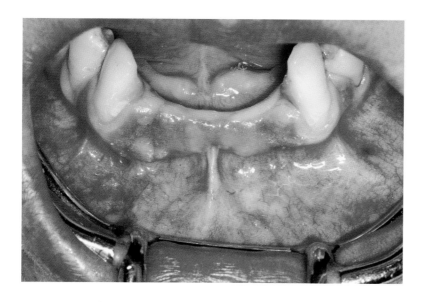

Fig 3-28 (a) Width defect at the anterior mandible. Again bone will be harvested from the vicinity avoiding morbidity at distant sites.

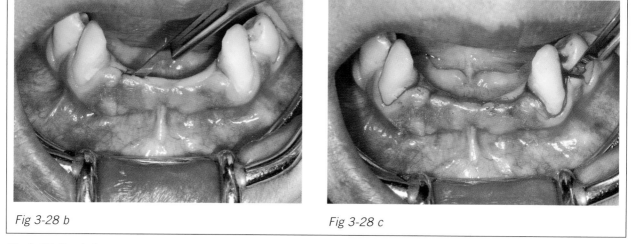

Fig 3-28 b

Fig 3-28 c

Fig 3-28 (b, c) Crestal and sulcular incisions.

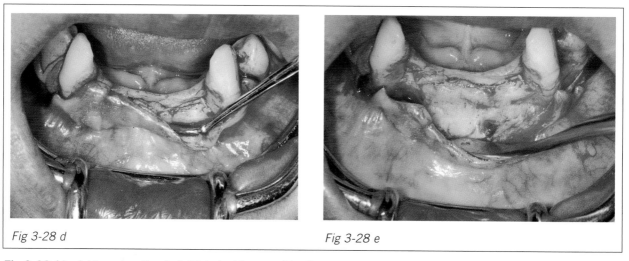

Fig 3-28 d

Fig 3-28 e

Fig 3-28 (d, e) Flap elevation is initiated with a papilla dissector and continued with a periosteal elevator.

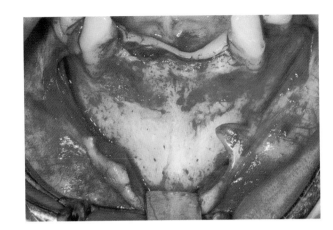

Fig 3-28 (f) Two relieving incisions are made at teeth 34 and 43 respectively. Insertion of the mucosa is preserved at tooth 44 so as not to further compromise its periodontal status.

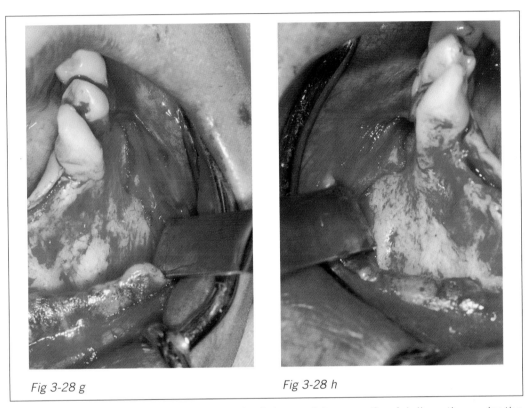

Fig 3-28 g

Fig 3-28 h

Fig 3-28 (g, h) These images depict the exit of the mental nerves. Careful dissection under the periosteal layer prevents neural injury.

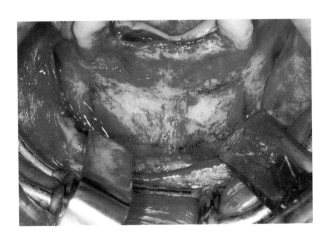

Fig 3-28 (i) Design of the graft according to the defect to be reconstructed is done with a wax pencil.

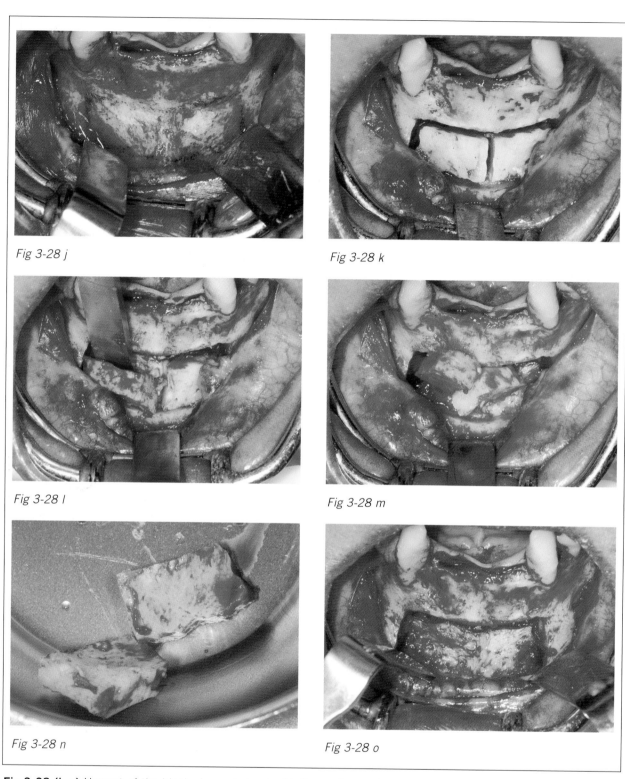

Fig 3-28 j

Fig 3-28 k

Fig 3-28 l

Fig 3-28 m

Fig 3-28 n

Fig 3-28 o

Fig 3-28 (j, o) Harvest of the blocks is carried out with fissure bur and chisel.

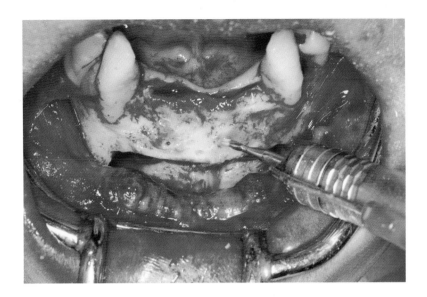

Fig 3-28 (p) 'Activation' of the recipient site is achieved by making holes in the cortex, thus facilitating medullary invasion of the graft.

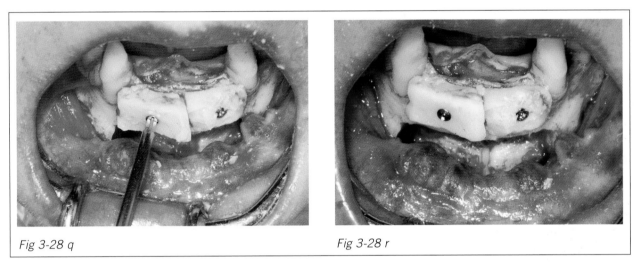

Fig 3-28 q

Fig 3-28 r

Fig 3-28 (q, r) Graft fixation correcting AP dimensions of the crest.

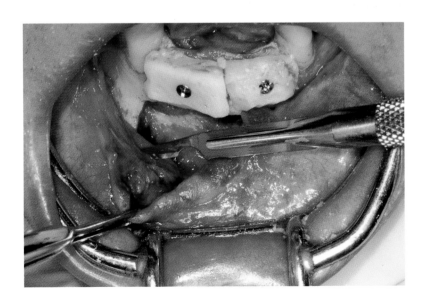

Fig 3-28 (s) Relieving incisions in the periosteum facilitate covering the reconstruction.

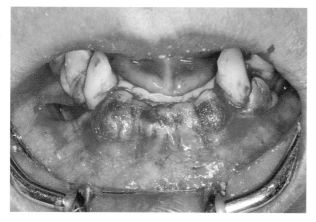

Fig 3-28 (t) Suturing starts at the critical area - in this case, the crest.

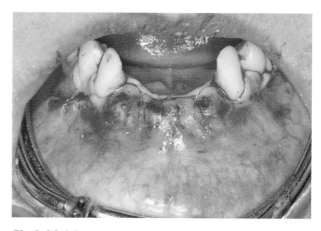

Fig 3-28 (u) Lateral incisions are closed next.

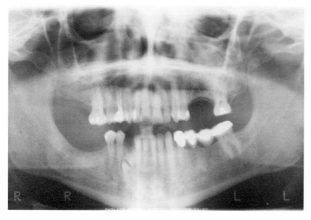

Fig 3-29 (a) Inferior right cuspid impacted because of the presence of an odontoma.

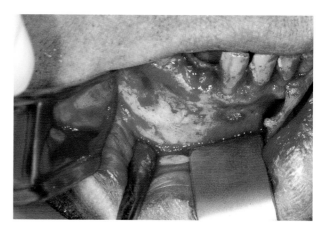

Fig 3-29 (b) Sulcular and crestal incision followed by subperiosteal dissection.

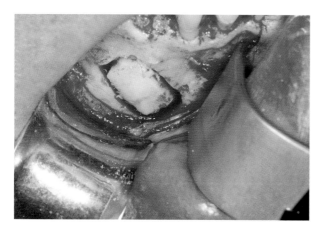

Fig 3-29 (c) A bone window is designed to gain access so that it will eventually be used as a bone graft.

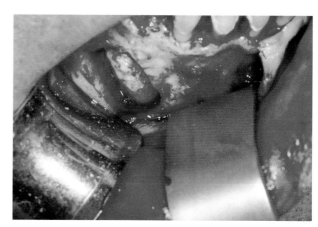

Fig 3-29 (d) The cuspid is uncovered.

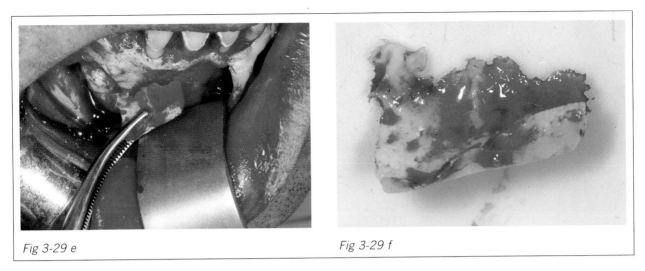

Fig 3-29 e

Fig 3-29 f

Fig 3-29 (e, f) Cortical graft.

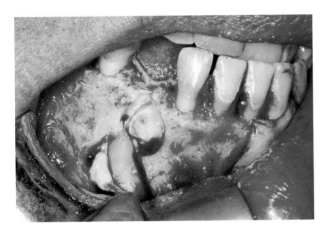

Fig 3-29 (g) Further uncovering of the odontoma reveals the size of the future defect.

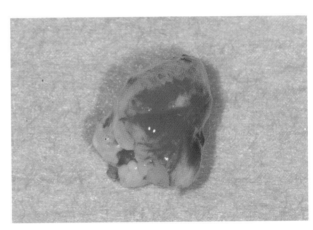

Fig 3-29 (h) Odontoma following removal.

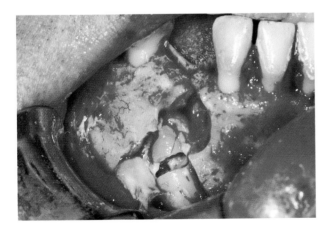

Fig 3-29 (i) Dividing the cuspid facilitates removal.

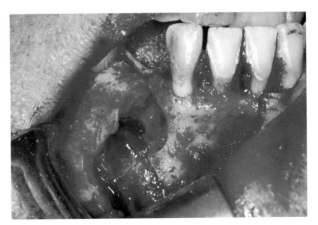

Fig 3-29 (j) Once the odontoma and cuspid have been removed the tri-dimensional aspect of the defect can be evaluated.

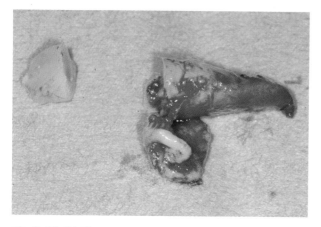

Fig 3-29 (k) The sectioned cuspid and follicle.

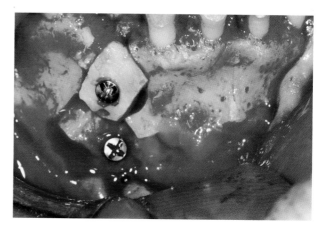

Fig 3-29 (l) The cortical window together with another piece from the chin allow reconstruction of the defect.

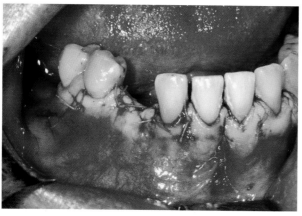

Fig 3-29 (m) Closing of the flap with repositioning of the papillae.

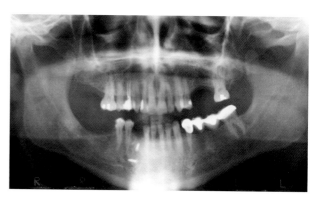

Fig 3-29 (n) Control panoramic X-ray.

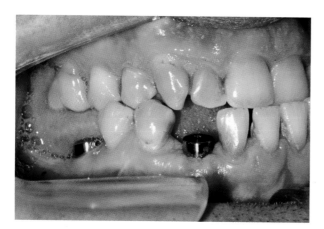

Fig 3-29 (o) Fixture placement three months after reconstruction.

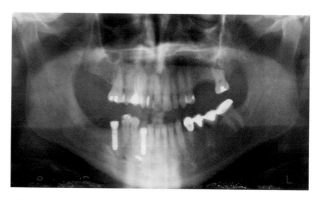

Fig 3-29 (p) Post-fixture panoramic X-ray. Note how the lower screw has been left in place, since it did not disturb fixture insertion.

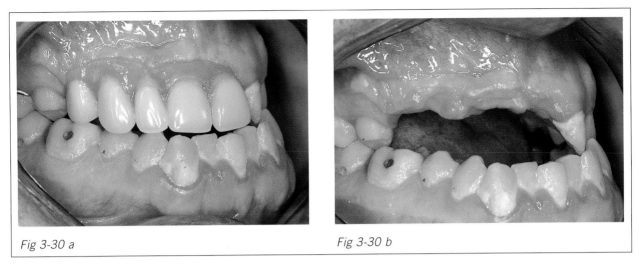

Fig 3-30 a   Fig 3-30 b

Fig 3-30 (a, b) Traumatic avulsion of an antero-lateral segment in a patient with a previous class III malocclusion and open bite. Vertical reconstruction of the crest is needed to allow proper positioning of the fixtures. Note the good quality and quantity of the soft tissues at the alveolar crest. On-lay or saddle grafts in this area give unpleasant aesthetic results because of the impairment in soft tissues. Every effort should be made in the aesthetic zone to preserve keratinised mucosa attached to the crest.

Fig 3-30 (c) A segmental osteotomy is planned to allow reduction of the defective zone without disturbing the crest. A high vestibular incision is recommended.

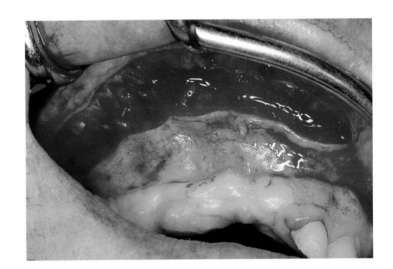

Fig 3-30 (d) Osteotomy design is achieved using a reciprocating saw.

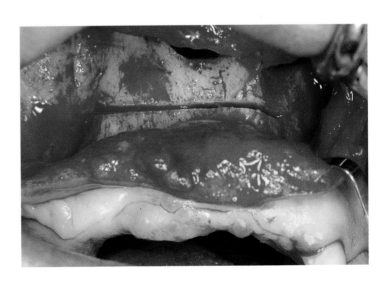

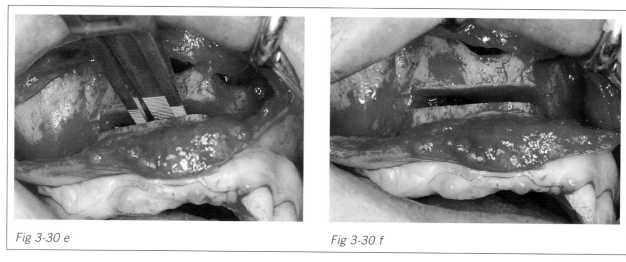

Fig 3-30 e
Fig 3-30 f

Fig 3-30 (e, f) A bone spreader is then used to move the segment vertically to the planned position.

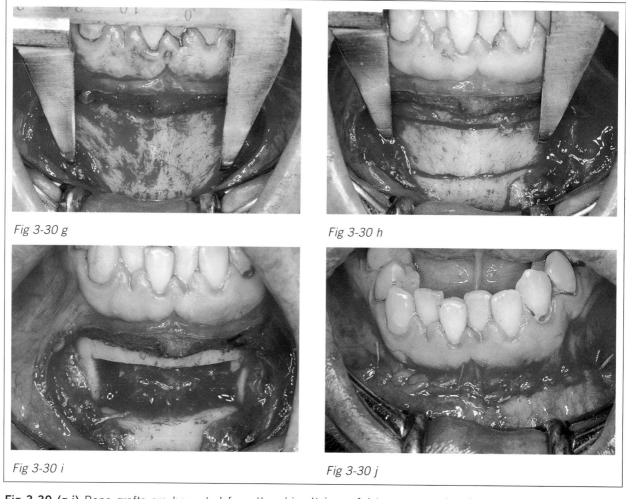

Fig 3-30 g
Fig 3-30 h

Fig 3-30 i
Fig 3-30 j

Fig 3-30 (g-j) Bone grafts are harvested from the chin. It is useful to measure the size of the grafts required to accurately harvest according to needs.

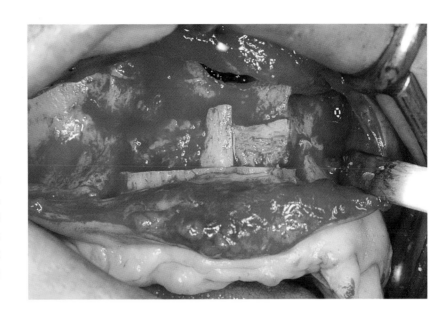

Fig 3-30 (k) Blocks from the chin are placed as interpositional grafts, maintaining the segment in the desired vertical position. No fixation is needed, since the blocks are kept in place due to the pressure from the segment.

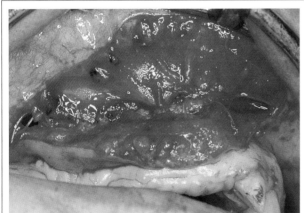

Fig 3-30 l

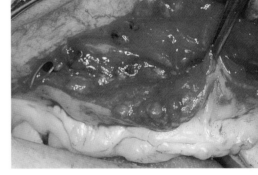

Fig 3-30 m

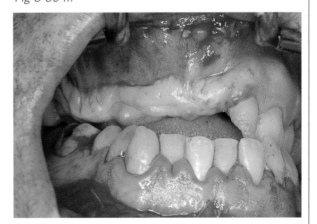

Fig 3-30 (l-n) Closure is achieved in two layers to protect the reconstruction and minimise scarring. The first layer is the periosteum and muscle, the second layer the mucosa.

Fig 3-30 n

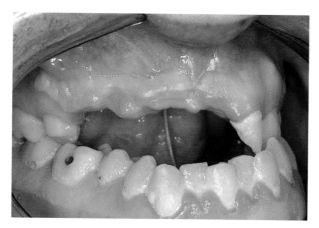

Fig 3-30 (o) Initial situation compared with the previous image.

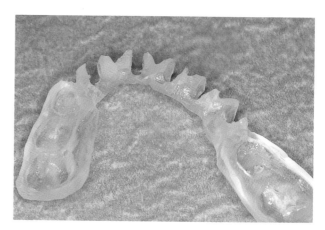

Fig 3-30 (p) Surgical stent to allow placement of the implants four months later.

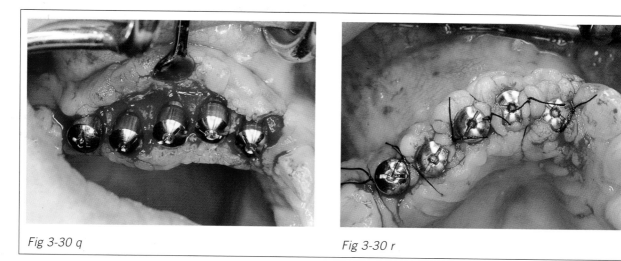

Fig 3-30 q   *Fig 3-30 r*

Fig 3-30 (q, r) Fixture placement and abutment connection at a single stage. Note the quality of tissues surrounding the implants. This kind of result is difficult to achieve when a crestal approach is used with onlay or saddle grafts. In addition, this situation is more prone to graft exposure.

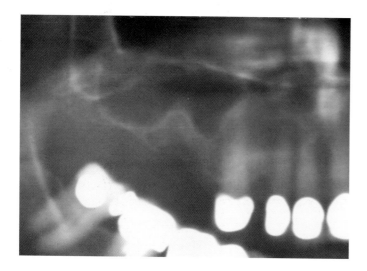

Fig 3-31 (a) Posterior maxillary atrophy. Use of bone blocks allows immediate insertion of fixtures, which act as fixation screws. Panoramic X-ray depicts residual height of the crest as well as the presence of a small septum in the sinus floor.

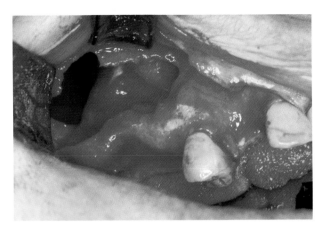

Fig 3-31 (b) Surgical approach to the sinus. The access window should be big enough to allow placement of the graft.

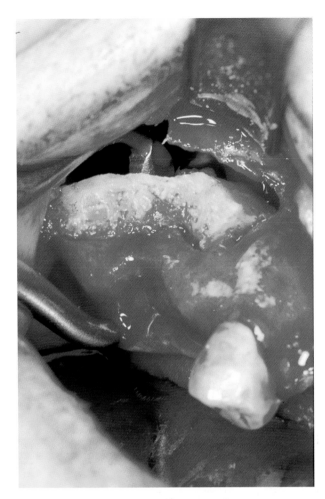

Fig 3-31 (c) Adaptation of a chin graft to the irregularities of the sinus floor.

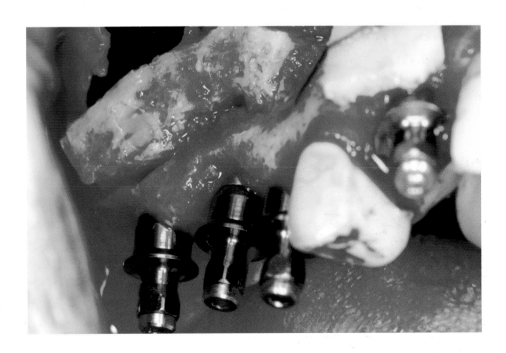

Fig 3-31 (d) Immediate placement of fixtures.

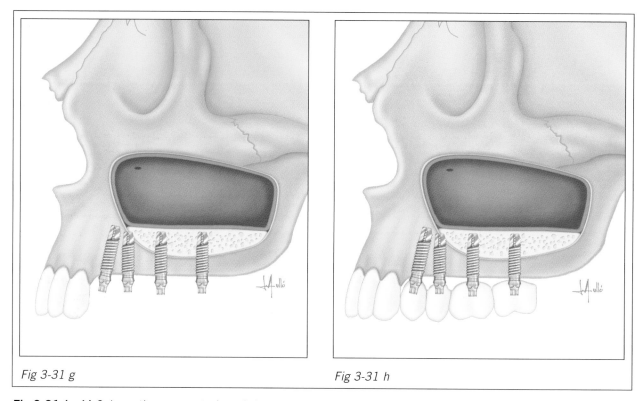

Fig 3-31 e *Fig 3-31 f*

Fig 3-31 (e, f) Final prosthetic result. This type of approach allows full reconstruction in a single stage.

Fig 3-31 g *Fig 3-31 h*

Fig 3-31 (g, h) Schematic representation of the procedure.

References

1   Garg AK, Morales MJ, Navarro I, Duarte F. Autogenous mandibular bone grafts in the treatment of the resorbed maxillary anterior alveolar ridge: Rationale and approach. Implant Dent 1998;7:169-176.

2   Citardi MJ, Friedman CD. Nonvascularized autogenous bone grafts for craniofacial skeletal augmentation and replacement. Otolaryngol Clin North Am 1994;27:891-910.

3   Jensen J, Simonsen EK, Sindet Pedersen S. Reconstruction of the severely resorbed maxilla with bone grafting and osseointegrated implants: A preliminary report. J Oral Maxillofacial Surg 1990;48:27-32.

4   Lundgren S, Moy P, Johansson C, Nilsson H. Augmentation of the maxillary sinus floor with particulated mandible: A histologic and histomorphometric study. Int J Oral Maxillofac Implants 1996;11:760-766.

5   Wood RM, Moore DL. Grafting of the maxillary sinus with intraorally harvested autogenous bone prior to implant placement. Int J Oral Maxillofac Implants 1988;3:209-213.

6   Hoppenreijs TJM, Nijdam ES, Freihofer HPM. The chin as a donor site in early secondary osteoplasty: A retrospective clinical and radiological evaluation. J Craniomaxillofac Surg 1992;20:119-124.

7   Misch CM. Comparison of intraoral donor sites for onlay grafting prior to implant placement. Int J Oral Maxillofac Implants 1997;12:767-776.

8   Misch CM, Misch CE. The repair of localized severe ridge defects for implant placement using mandibular bone grafts. Implant Dent 1995;4:261-267.

9   Triplett RG, Schow SR. Autologous bone grafts and endosseous implants: Complementary techniques. J Oral Maxillofac Surg 1996;54:486-534.

10 Nystrom E, Legrell PE, Forsell A, Kahnberg KE. Combined use of bone grafts and implants in the severely resorbed maxilla. Int J Oral Maxillofac Surg 1995;24:20-25.

11 Borstlap WA, Heidbuchel K, Freihofer HPM, Kuijpers-Jagtman AM. Early secondary bone grafting of alveolar cleft defects: A comparison between chin and rib grafts. J Craniomaxillofac Surg 1990;18:201-205.

12 Kusiak JF, Zins JE, Whitaker LA. The early revascularization of membranous bone. Plast Reconstr Surg 1985;76:510-516.

13 Smith JD, Abramson M: Membraneous vs. endochondral bone autografts. Arch Otolaryngol 1974;99:203.

14 Zins JE, Whitaker LA: Membraneous vs endochondral bone autografts: Implications for craniofacial reconstruction. Surg Form 1979;30:521.

15 Misch CE: Density of bone: Effect on treatment plans, surgical approach, healing and progressive bone loading. Int J Oral Implantol 1990;6:23-31.

16 Johansson B, Wannfors K, Ekenbäck J, Smedberg JI, Hirsch J. Implants and sinus-inlay bone grafts in a 1-stage procedure on severely atrophied maxillae: Surgical aspects of a 3-year follow-up study. Int J Oral Maxillofac Implants 1999;14:811-818.

17 Listrom RD, Symington JS: Osseointegrated dental implants in conjunction with bone grafts. Int J Oral Maxillofac Surg 1988;17:116-118.

18 Montazem A, Valauri DV, St-Hilaire H et al. The mandibular symphysis as a donor site in maxillofacial bone grafting: A quantitative anatomic study. J Oral Maxillofac Surg 2000;58:1368.

19 McCarthy C, Patel RR, Wragg PF, Brook IM. Dental implants and onlay bone grafts in the anterior maxilla: Analysis and clinical outcome. Int J Oral Maxillofac Implants 2003;18:238-241.

20 Widmark G, Andersson B, Ivanoff CJ. Mandibular bone graft in the anterior maxilla for single-tooth implants. Presentation of a surgical method. Int J Oral Maxillofac Surg 1997;26:106-109.

21 Raghoebar GM, Batenburg RH, Vissenk A, Reintsema H. Augmentation of localized defects on the anterior maxillary ridge with autogenous bone before insertion of implants. J Oral Maxillofac Surg 1996;54:1180-1185.

Chapter 4

Ascending Ramus and Body

Surgical Anatomy

Bone grafts from the body and ascending ramus of the mandible exhibit similar behaviour to those from the chin. They share a common embryologic origin (first and second branchial archs). Being membranous, they also have a slower resorption rate.[1-5] One important difference between chin and body and ramus grafts is the fact that the inferior alveolar nerve lies under the latter. At least theoretically, the chances of injuring the bundle are higher in these posterior areas (Fig 4-1 a, b).

Body of the mandible

These grafts can be harvested from an area limited anteriorly by the mental foramen and posteriorly by the third molar area (Fig 4-2a). The amount of available bone depends largely on

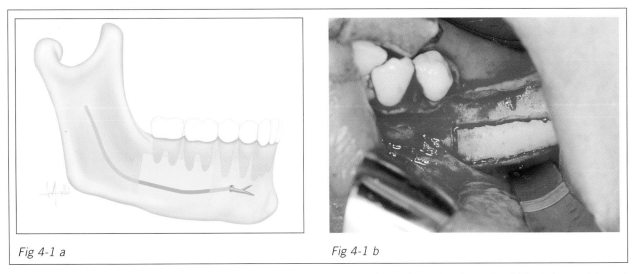

Fig 4-1 a

Fig 4-1 b

Fig 4-1 (a, b) The inferior alveolar nerve lies beneath the donor area for body grafts. Care should be taken not to cut beyond the cortical plate at this level.

age, gender and degree of mandibular atrophy. Li and Schwartz determined that the average bone size obtained from the lateral plate of the mandibular body was 13x30mm (Fig 4-2 a, b).[6]

The width of the graft is limited by the presence of the inferior alveolar bundle, which obviously constitutes the deep limit of the graft. In most cases grafts from this area are made of a dense monocortical bone. Little or no cancellous bone can be harvested.

Ascending ramus

This area is limited inferiorly by the retromolar region, superiorly by the coronoid process and sigmoid notch, and posteriorly by the entrance of the inferior alveolar bundle at the level of the Spix spine.

According to Güngörmüs[7] the average dimensions of the grafts obtained from this area are 37.60x33.17x22.48x9.15mm, 2.36ml being the average bone volume and the average surface area being 495.13mm². However, in this study the coronoid process was also included. Without it, in our experience, the length of the graft is reduced to approx 25mm.

The thickness and morphology of the bone graft harvested from this region is not homogeneous. The width of the ascending ramus diminishes when ascending towards the sigmoid notch, and at this level both cortical layers fuse.

When considering the ascending ramus as a donor site a careful radiological study, preferably with the aid of a CT scan, is encouraged, to avoid damaging the inferior alveolar neurovascular bundle.

Qualitatively, grafts from the ascending ramus are monocortical with little or no cancellous bone.

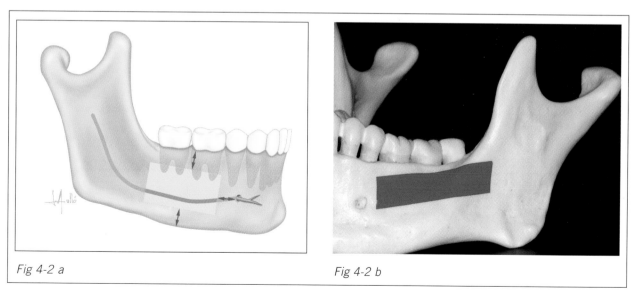

Fig 4-2 a

Fig 4-2 b

Fig 4-2 (a, b) The rule of '5s' also applies in this area. A 5mm margin should be left from the exit of the bundle, the inferior mandibular border and the neck of the bicuspids and molars.

Surgical Procedure

Procurement of grafts from the body and ramus of the mandible can be done under local anaesthesia. In selected cases intravenous sedation can be used, but in all cases a vasoconstrictor agent will reduce blood loss.

Anaesthesia

This should be infiltrative in the molar and bicuspid region. We prefer not to block the inferior alveolar nerve in order to have an alarm mechanoceptive system in case we approach the mandibular canal.

Access

An intrasulcular incision to minimise periosteal tears is undertaken from the second bicuspid to the retromolar area. In edentulous patients it should be prepared at the alveolar crest. A posterior vestibular-relieving incision is needed in most cases (Fig 4-3 a-d).

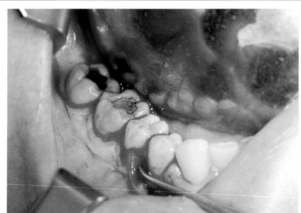

Fig 4-3 a

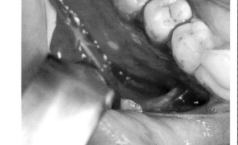

Fig 4-3 b

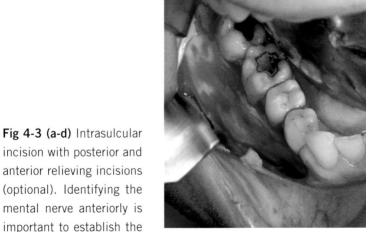

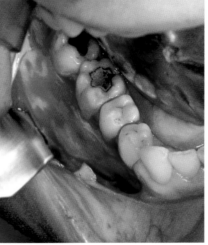

Fig 4-3 (a-d) Intrasulcular incision with posterior and anterior relieving incisions (optional). Identifying the mental nerve anteriorly is important to establish the anterior limit of the graft.

Fig 4-3 c

Fig 4-3 d

Careful subperiosteal dissection is carried out with a sharp periosteal elevator to avoid damaging the neurovascular bundle where it exits the mental foramen.

Harvesting procedure

To proceed safely to the donor area, the '5s' rule should be followed just like at the symphyseal region, staying 5mm away from mental foramen, inferior border of the mandible. However, instead of staying 5mm under the roots, the reference in this case are the necks of the neighbouring crowns or the uppermost line of the crest, respectively. This is due to the increased width of the mandibular body at this level (Fig 4-4). Here, in addition, we must bear in mind that the mandibular canal lies under our planned graft. To avoid it a careful radiological analysis is essential.

Different methods of graft procurement can be used, depending on the required amount of bone and the size of the defect.

When corticocancellous blocks are needed, careful analysis of the recipient or defective area should be done to match the amount of bone grafted to the actual needs.

When harvesting at the mandibular body, osteotomies should be corticotomies to avoid invading the canal and severing the neurovascular bundle.

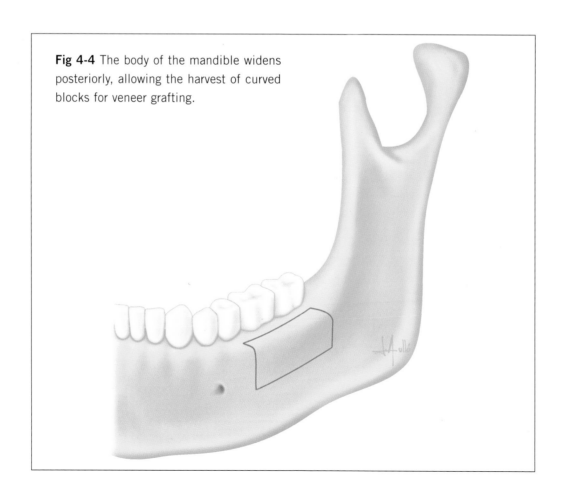

Fig 4-4 The body of the mandible widens posteriorly, allowing the harvest of curved blocks for veneer grafting.

The choice of instruments at this stage is as follows:

- Fissure bur (No. 702) - a cheap, very effective instrument. Provides very sensitive control of the cut and makes a wide enough groove to allow further positioning of the chisel (Fig 4-5a).
- Saw-preferably an oscillating one. Makes thin cuts that should be convergent (extrusive) (Fig 4-5 b, c).
- Disk - acts as a saw, making very thin cuts. It is essential to have a guard to protect soft tissues. Even when protected it is a dangerous instrument and unless carefully controlled the chances of damaging surrounding tissues are high.

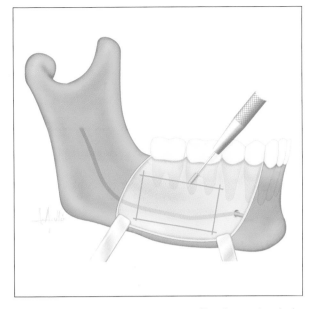

Fig 4-5 (a) Fissure burs are very effective and safe in designing the cuts at this level.

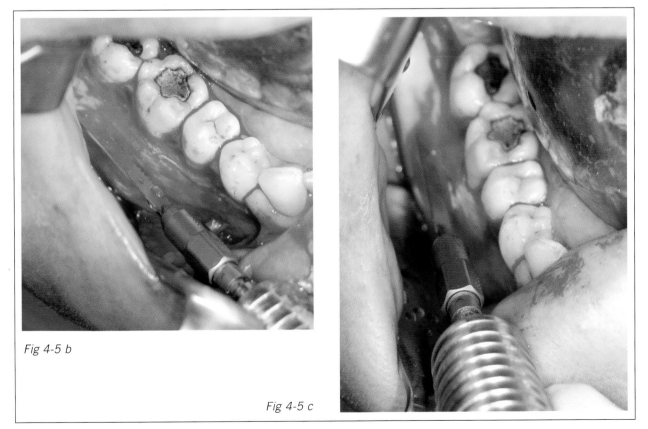

Fig 4-5 b

Fig 4-5 c

Fig 4-5 (b, c) Thin saws are a good, albeit expensive, alternative. The advantage of using the saw is minimal trauma due to the fine cut. Disadvantage is less feeling when crossing the cortical plate.

- Trephines - indicated when small cores of corticocancellous bone are needed. Depending on the trephine, diameter cores may range between 4-10mm. When using a trephine, it is important to remain clear – over or under – of the imaginary projected pattern of the canal at the surface.

In most cases the desired block will be a monocortical one. The scarce cancellous bone in the area surrounds the mandibular canal and should be avoided.

As in the previous chapter regarding the chin, once the osteotomy has been designed, a sharp chisel will be inserted in the crease and carefully bent to allow dislodgement of the block (Fig 4-6 a-c).

Before performing the osteotomies, careful planning of the reconstructive needs has to be completed in order to avoid over or under-harvesting. Due to the cephalo-caudal convexity of the mandible at this level, the inferior cortico-tomy is quite difficult to perform. An angled

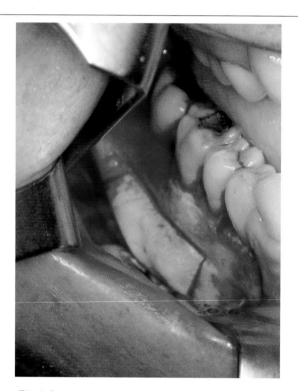

Fig 4-6 a

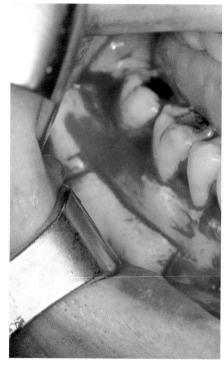

Fig 4-6 b

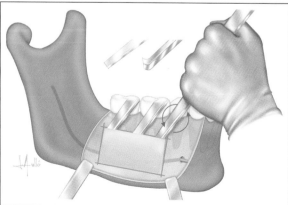

Fig 4-6 c

Fig 4-6 (a-c) Once the osteotomy has been designed, bending curved chisels in the superior groove detaches the block.

hand piece with a guarded disk or an oscillating saw will help at this stage.

Split of the graft from the donor site should be carried out with care with the aid of curved and straight osteotomes. Limited force should be applied to reduce the risk of bad splitting of the graft and/or fracturing the mandible. To avoid this the osteotomy pattern must be checked and it must be clear that the osteotomies have gone through the cortical plate at all sites. The graft should be split as a single unit and if it requires division into further pieces this should be done extraorally. In this way we avoid performing additional vertical osteotomies thus reducing the risk of encountering the neurovascular bundle. Using a mallet on the osteotomes at this site is forbidden in order to avoid trauma to the temporomandibular joint and because of the risk of entering the medullary bone and severing the bundle.

When beginning to harvest grafts from the body of the mandible, it is advisable to use diamond burs in order to prevent damaging the bundle in the event that one runs into the canal.

When separating the graft from the mandible we occasionally find the bundle adhering to the graft. Should this be the case, a blunt nerve dissector should be used to replace it. Often, after removing the graft, it is possible to pinpoint the location of the neurovascular bundle. If further cancellous bone needs to be harvested, care should be taken to avoid neural damage (Fig 4-7 a-c).

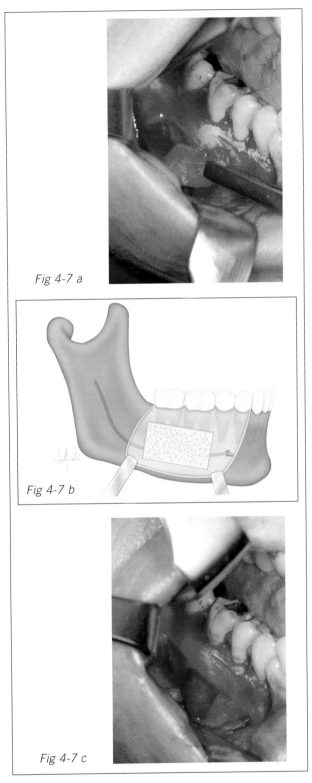

Fig 4-7 a

Fig 4-7 b

Fig 4-7 c

Fig 4-7 (a-c) After the block has been removed, extra cancellous bone can be harvested, with care not to damage the bundle. Magnification and blunt curettes are useful.

Once removed, the graft should be protected by humid gauze until it is positioned at the recipient site.

Suturing begins with the repositioning of the relieving incisions with 5/0 resorbable material and continues with papillae adequately repositioned with transpapillary sutures (Fig 4-8).

Mandibular ramus

Anatomical references are also important when considering a ramus harvest (Fig 9 a, b).

Harvesting of a ramus graft should be done under local anaesthesia, with infiltration in the retromolar area over the bone as well as laterally and medially.

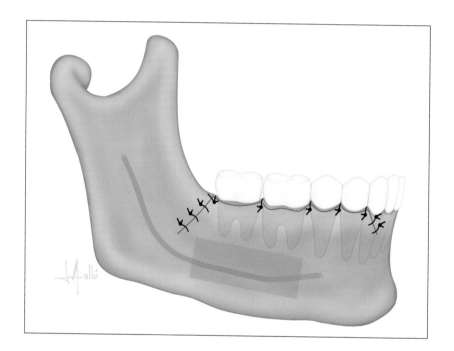

Fig 4-8 Interrupted sutures are used to reposition the flap.

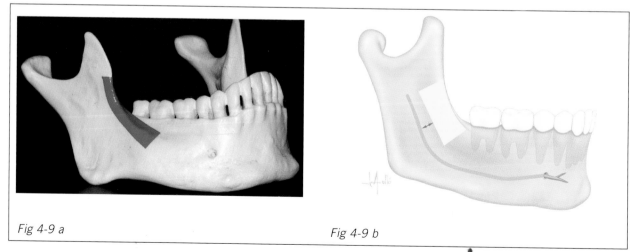

Fig 4-9 a

Fig 4-9 b

Fig 4-9 (a, b) Observing anatomical limits of the ramus region is important to avoid injury of neural structures.

A vertical through-and-through incision of 20mm is made either with a No. 15 blade or with a fine needle connected to a surgical knife (for instance, a Colorado needle). In both cases the incision should be carried down to the bone approx 10mm over the mandibular alveolar crest. When performing the incision, palpation of the anterior border of the ascending ramus is essential to avoid deviations to the lingual side that might cause trauma to the lingual or the inferior alveolar nerves (Fig 4-9 c-e).

Dissection should then proceed with a sharp periosteal elevator peeling both periosteum and tendinous insertions from the temporalis muscle up from the bone. Often we find it necessary to use the scalpel to release some deep tendinous insertions from the bone. Should this be the case, peeling off these fibrous remnants from the graft is recommended. To ease the harvesting procedure we recommend retraction of the muscular and tendinous insertions with a curved bone clamp (Fig 4-9f).

Fig 4-9 (c-e) Palpation of the anterior crest aids in placing the incision right into the bone, thus avoiding the lingual or buccal nerves.

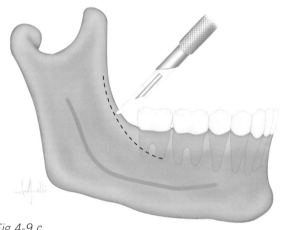

Fig 4-9 c

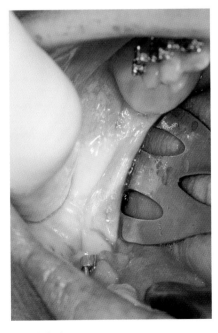

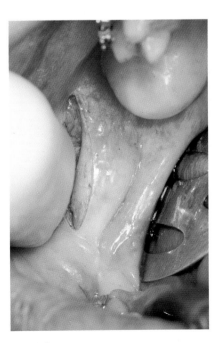

Fig 4-9 d

Fig 4-9 e

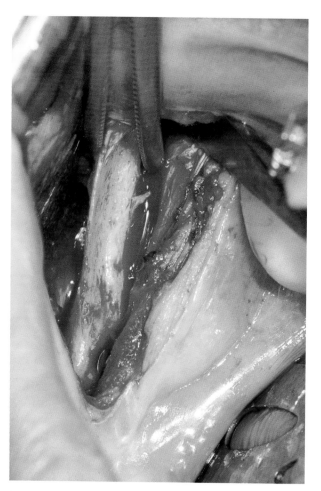

It is of outmost importance to proceed under the periosteum medially until the Spix spine is found and the entrance of the neurovascular bundle identified. This constitutes the posterior limit of our graft.

Corticotomies can be done with the same instruments recommended for the mandibular body. A diamond fissure bur with an angled hand piece is particularly useful in this case, due to the good control it offers. Experienced surgeons might find the use of a saw more efficient and fast. In this case both oscillating and reciprocating saws could be used (Fig 4-10a).

Again, separation of the graft from the ramus can be done by twisting an osteotome inserted in one of the grooves (Fig 4-10b) or, when the graft is small, by grasping it with a bone rongeur.

Fig 4-9 (f) After peeling tendinous insertions, a bone clamp aids in protecting soft tissues, clearing the bone for further osteotomies

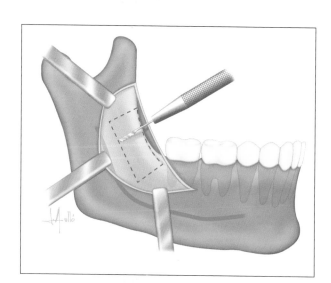

Fig 4-10 (a) A reciprocating saw is useful in designing the horizontal cuts.

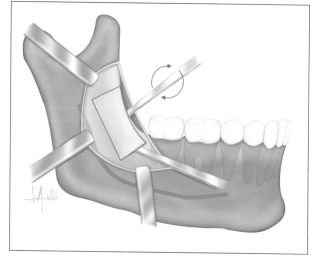

Fig 4-10 (b) Dislodgement of the graft is easily done with a chisel.

Occasionally we may see the bundle after removal of the graft,[8,9] but in most instances we will stay away from the canal (Fig 4-11).

A 5/0 running suture will allow fast and effective closure of the incision (Fig 4-12).

Clinical Applications

The use of monocortical grafts from the mandibular body and ramus is especially indicated for veneer grafting in different areas. Small to moderate width defects are easily managed with this 'friendly' graft.

When mild (less than 5mm) vertical defects of the alveolar crest are present, this donor site can also be of use.[10]

Although beyond the scope of this book, different applications for maxillofacial reconstruction have been proposed.[11-14]

Ramus grafts are often suitable as saddle grafts or 'J' grafts to correct small vertical and vestibulo-lingual defects of the crest (Fig 4-13 a-f).

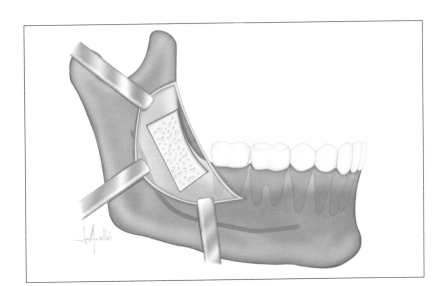

Fig 4-11 Accurate design of the osteotomies should avoid the bundle duct.

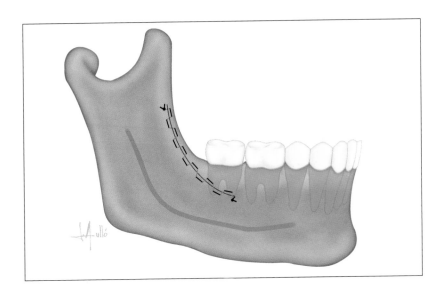

Fig 4-12 Running 5/0 resorbable sutures should approach both the muscle and the mucosa.

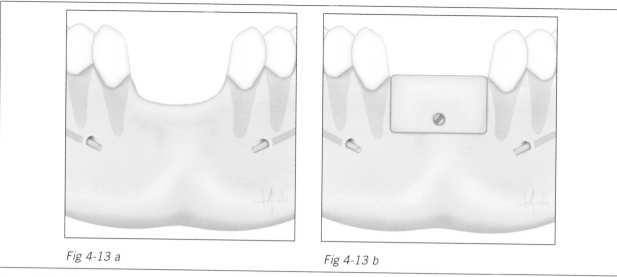

Fig 4-13 a   *Fig 4-13 b*

Fig 4-13 (a, b) Onlay and veneer grafting are common indications for body and ramus harvesting.

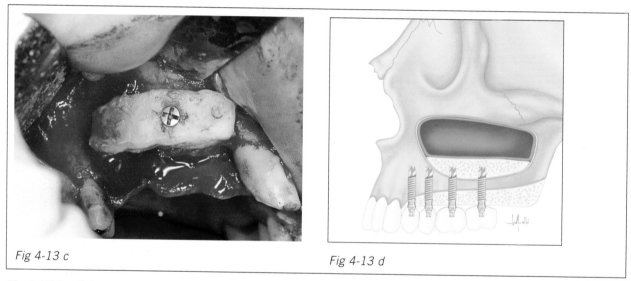

Fig 4-13 c   *Fig 4-13 d*

Fig 4-13 (c, d) Crestal onlay grafting at the posterior maxilla to normalise crestal height, and simultaneous insertion of fixtures.

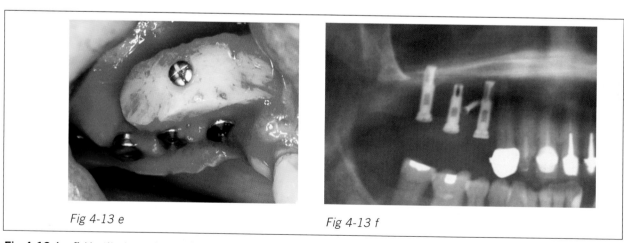

Fig 4-13 e   *Fig 4-13 f*

Fig 4-13 (e, f) Vestibular onlay grafting at the posterior maxilla and immediate implant insertion.

Another advantage of this donor site is the fact of having two sites on each mandible, thus allowing 'double' harvesting from any given patient.

Quite often we use body and ramus grafts for vertical or transverse defects in the posterior mandible (Fig 4-14 a-g). The possibility of having donor and receptor sites within the same surgical site is cost – effective and obviously decreases morbidity and postoperative disturbances.

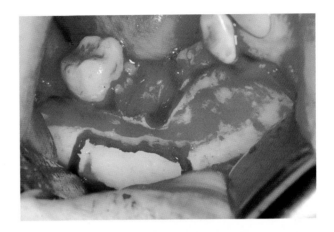

Fig 4-14 (a) Vestibular defect at the bicuspid area in the mandible. The first molar has been removed because of root fracture. A body graft is designed to correct the transverse defect. Note how the '5s' rule is applied, placing the upper osteotomy 5mm away from the neighbouring crowns. The cancellous bone is seen through the grooves if corticotomy is adequately performed.

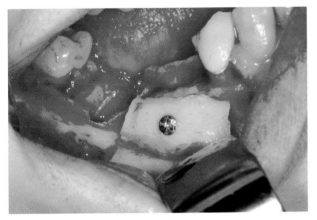

Fig 4-14 (b) Graft fixation with compression screw restoring crestal dimensions.

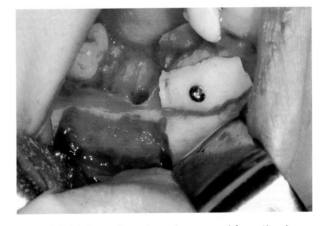

Fig 4-14 (c) Cancellous bone is removed from the donor site to fill the space in the alveolus left by the extracted molar.

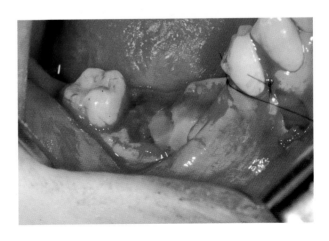

Fig 4-14 (d) PRP keeps the particulated bone in place while suturing.

97

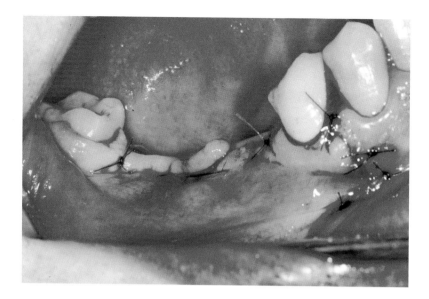

Fig 4-14 (e) 5/0 interrupted sutures are used, everting flap edges. Extra-advancement of the flap is achieved through periosteal incisions, thus allowing closure without tension in the molar area.

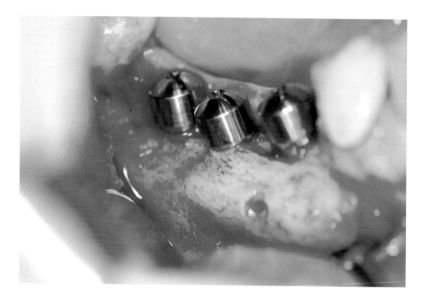

Fig 4-14 (f) Re-entry three months after the procedure reveals adequate healing of bone grafts, thus allowing fixture placement and screw removal.

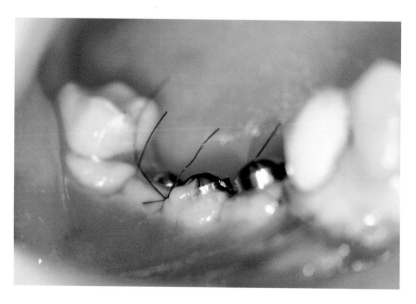

Fig 4-14 (g) Abutment connection at same surgery.

The recipient site should be 'activated' to allow for faster incorporation of the graft.[15,16,17] This is easily achieved by creating small holes with a fissure bur and thus allowing communication between the medullary space of the recipient site and the deep surface of the graft. Again, rigid fixation of the graft is essential, and a single compression screw will suffice (Fig 15, 16, 17).

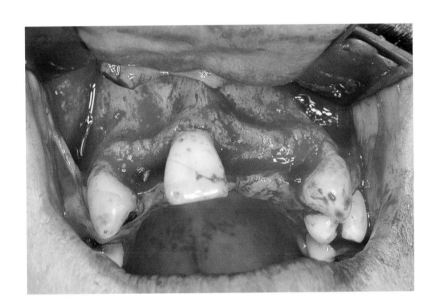

Fig 4-15 Vestibular defects at the anterior maxilla due to disuse.

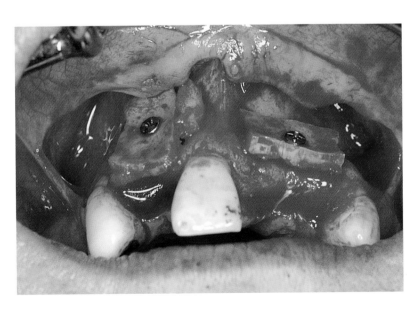

Fig 4-16 Veneer reconstruction with cortical pieces obtained from the ramus.

99

Fig 4-17 a

Fig 4-17 b

Fig 4-17 c

Fig 4-17 d

Fig 4-17 (a-d) Traumatic avulsion of three upper incisors together with buccal bone, leaving a transversely deficient crest.

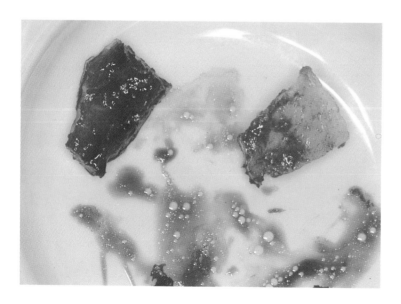

Fig 4-17 (e) Two pieces of cortical bone are harvested from the body of the mandible.

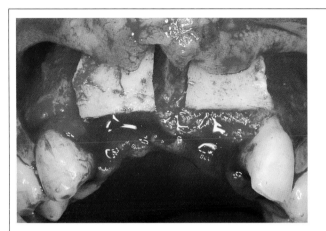

Fig 4-17 f

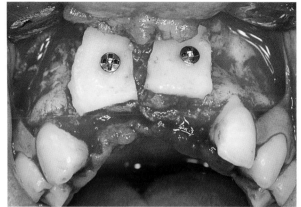

Fig 4-17 g

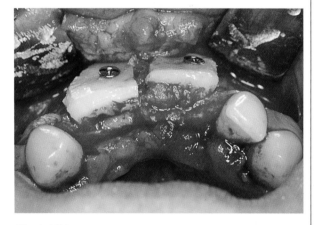

Fig 4-17 h

Fig 4-17 (f-h) Graft trimming, adaptation and fixation for adequate reconstruction.

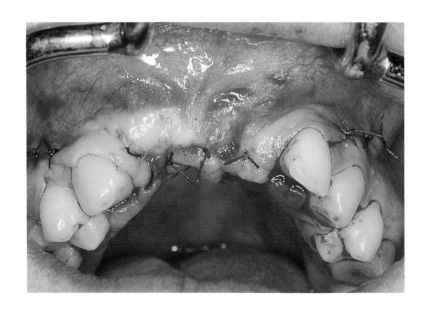

Fig 4-17 (i) Eversion of the flaps and suture with interrupted 5/0.

Fig 4-17 j

Fig 4-17 k

Fig 4-17 (j, k) Post and pre-surgical status reveals 4mm vertical increase.

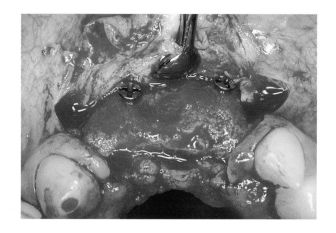

Fig 4-17 (l) Re-entry four months later showing remodelling and incorporation of the graft in the recipient site. Note how flap design preserves papillae and brings keratinised mucosa to the buccal side.

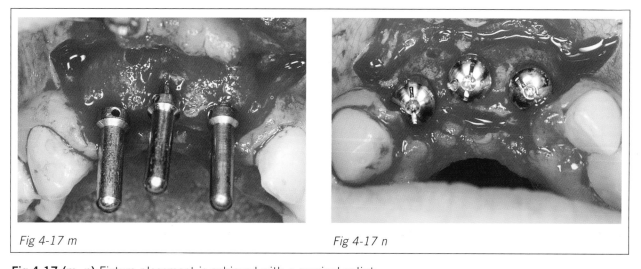

Fig 4-17 m

Fig 4-17 n

Fig 4-17 (m, n) Fixture placement is achieved with a surgical splint.

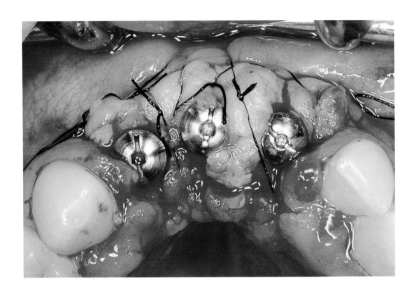

Fig 4-17 (o) Flap redistribution and tailoring around the abutments.

Often, in spite of a meticulous adaptation of the graft to the recipient site small spaces may persist between both. Small portions of particulated bone with PRP as carrier can be introduced in these spaces to eliminate the risk of fibrous in-growth (Fig 18 a-g). A watertight suture without tension will prevent suture dehiscences.[18,19]

103

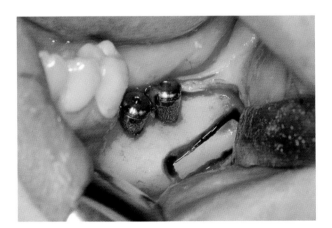

Fig 4-18 (a) Two fixtures placed in the posterior mandible, leaving a vestibular fenestration. A small block from the ramus is designed without changing or modifying the surgical field. Osteotomy is carried out with a fissure bur.

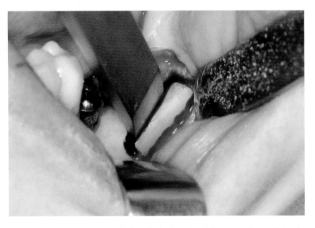

Fig 4-18 (b) The graft is dislodged with a wedge chisel.

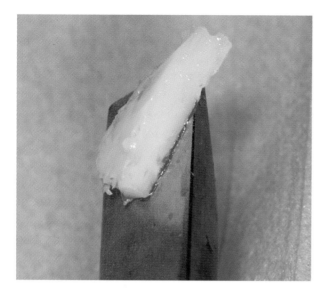

Fig 4-18 (c) Note how the graft is made exclusively of cortical bone.

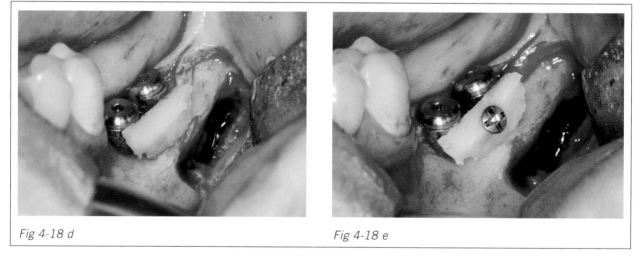

Fig 4-18 d   Fig 4-18 e

Fig 4-18 (d, e) Positioning and fixing of the graft with a compression screw.

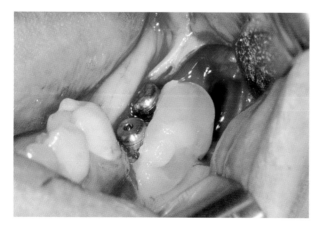

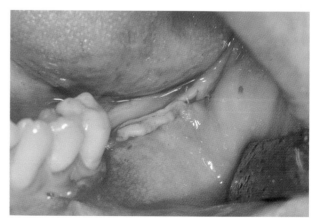

Fig 4-18 (f) Extra bone chips from the donor site are harvested and placed between the fixtures. A PRP membrane is positioned, covering the graft.

Fig 4-18 (g) Eversion of the flaps is maintained with a resorbable 5/0 monofilament.

Complications

Intraoperatory

Neurovascular: The inferior alveolar bundle can be severed during the harvesting procedure either at its intraoseous part or once it has exited from the mental foramen.

Palpation of the anterior border of the ramus and keeping the incision on it will avoid severing of both the buccal and the lingual nerve.

Careful retraction of the flaps is also essential to avoid stretching of the nerves.

When dissecting the lower border of the mandibular body it is of utmost importance to keep a subperiosteal plane to avoid injuring ascending branches of the facial artery.

Dental: Disturbing dental apices can be avoided by using the 5mm rule and judicious evaluation of radiographs.

Mandibular fracture: Although this is a rare occurrence, if it happens immediate referral to an oral and maxillofacial surgery unit is required for rigid fixation with miniplates.

Postoperative

Swelling: Mild to moderate swelling can be anticipated, especially when harvesting from the ascending ramus. Disinsertion or cutting of muscle causes more pain and swelling. To avoid this we like to inject corticosteroids into the muscle.

Infection: To minimise the risk of infection we instigate prophylactic treatment with antibiotics pre-operatively and continue this for five days.

Neural: If the inferior alveolar nerve is exposed during surgery we can anticipate variable degrees of sensory disturbances during the postoperative period. Corticosteroids will help in accelerating the disinflamation process. The patient should be fully aware of this possibility before surgery, and this fact has to be incorporated to validate informed consent.

References

1 Jensen J, Sindet-Pedersen S. Autogenous mandibular bone grafts and osseointegrated implants for reconstruction of the severely atrophied maxilla: a preliminary report. J Oral Maxillofac Surg 1991;24:1277-1289.

2 Koole R, Bosker H, van der Dussen FU. Late secondary autogenous bone grafting in cleft patients comparing mandibular (ectomesenchymal) and iliac crest (mesenchymal) grafts. J Carniomaxillofac Surg 1989;17:28.

3 Smith JD, Abramsson M. Membranous vs endochondral bone autografts. Arch Laryngol 1974;99:203-205.

4 Zins JE, Whitaker LA. Membranous vs endochondral bone: Implications for craniofacial reconstruction. Plast Reconstr Surg 1983;72:778-784.

5 Kusiak JF, Zins JE, Whitaker LA. The early revascularization of membranous bone. Plast Reconstr Surg 1985,76:510-514.

6 Li KK, Schwartz HC. Mandibular body bone in facial plastic and reconstructive surgery. Laryngoscope 1996;106:504

7 Bedrossian E, Tawfilis A, Alijanian A. Veneer grafting: a technique for augmentation of the resorbed alveolus prior to implant placement. A clinical report. Int J Oral Maxillofac Implants 2000;15:853-858.

8 Güngörmüs M, Yavuz MS. The ascending ramus of the mandible as a donor site in maxillofacial bone grafting. J Oral Maxillofac Surg 2002;60:1316-1318.

9 Rajchel J, Ellis E III, Fonseca RJ. The anatomic location of the mandibular canal: its relationship to the sagital ramus osteotomy. Int J Adult Orthod Orthognath Surg 1986;1;37-47.

10 Proussaefs P, Lozada J, Kleinman A, Rohrer MD. The use of ramus autogenous block grafts for vertical alveolar ridge augmentation and implant placement: A pilot study. Int J Oral Maxillofac Implants 2002;17:238-248.

11 Muto T, Kanazawa M. Mandibular reconstruction using the anterior part of ascending ramus: Report of two cases. J Oral Maxillofac Surg 1997;55:1552.

12 Laskin JL, Edwards DM. Immediate reconstruction of an orbital complex fracture with autogenous mandibular bone. J Oral Surg 1977;35:749-751.

13 Lisa LY, Wijkie WK. Alternative donor site for alveolar bone grafting in adults with cleft lip and palate. Angle Orthodont 1996;6:9-12.

14 Sindet-Pedersen S, Enemark H. Mandibular bone grafts for reconstruction of alveolar clefts. J Oral Maxillofac Surg 1988;46:533.

15 Whitaker LA. Biological boundaries: A concept in facial skeletal restructuring. Clin Plast Surg 1989;16:1-10.

16 Rompen EH, Biewer R, Vanheusden A, et al. The influence of cortical perforations and of space filling with peripheral blood on the kinetics of guided bone regeneration. Clin Oral Implants Res 1999;10:85-94.

17 De Carvalho PS, Vasconcellos LW, Pi J. Influence of bed preparation on the incorporation of autogenous bone grafts: A study in dogs. Int J Oral Maxillofac Implants 2000;15:565-570.

18 Corn H. Periosteal separation: Its clinical significance. J Periodontol 1962;33:140-153.

19 Carranza FA, Carraro JJ, Dotto CA. Effect of periosteal fenestration in gingival extension operations. J Periodontol 1966;37:335-340.

Chapter 5 — Coronoid Process

Surgical Anatomy

The coronoid process (CP) (*processus coronoideus*) is located at the uppermost and anterior region of the mandibular ascending ramus. Transversely flat, it has a triangular shape. Its posterior edge constitutes the anterior limit of the sigmoid notch through which the masseteric artery and nerves wander. The coronoid process constitutes the main insertion of the temporalis muscle, which originates at the temporalis bone. This tendinous insertion is rigidly attached to both edges of the process and especially to the inner flat side.

As an important anatomical landmark, we must remember that the inferior alveolar nerve and artery enter the mandible medially only 10mm under the sigmoid notch.

Being part of the mandible, the CP is membranous in origin and formed by a thin layer of cancellous bone surrounded by two thick layers of dense cortical bone.

Its approximate dimensions are 2-3cm^2, 7-10mm wide at its base, and 2-3mm at its apex (Fig 5-1 a, b).

Surgical Technique

Harvesting of a CP graft should be carried out under local anaesthesia unless it is done as part of a more complex procedure.

A vertical through-and-through incision of 20mm is made either with a No. 15 blade or with a fine needle connected to a surgical knife (for instance, a Colorado needle). In both cases the incision should be carried down to the bone approx 10mm over the mandibular alveolar crest (Fig 5-2 a-d).

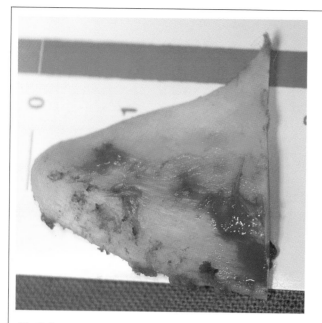

Fig 5-1 a

Fig 5-1 b

108

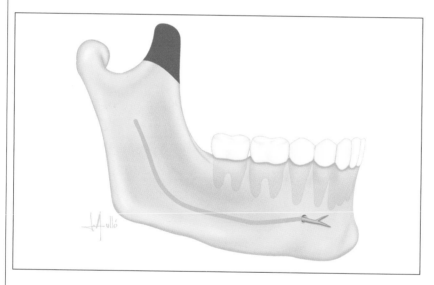

Fig 5-1 c

Fig 5-1 d

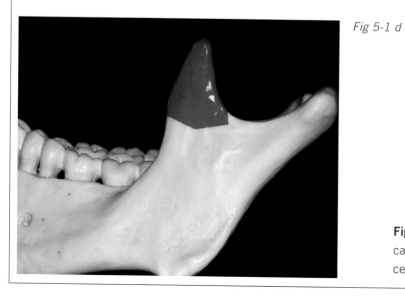

Fig 5-1 (a-d) Dimensions and anatomical limits of a standard coronoid process.

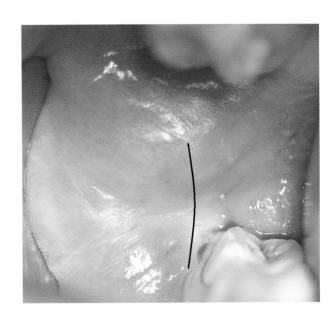

Fig 5-2 (a) The black line depicts location and size of the recommended incision for CP harvesting. Palpation with the index finger aids in locating the oblique line of the mandible.

Fig 5-2 (b-d) Incision proceeds through the muscle to reach the bone. Careful haemostasis is recommended at this point.

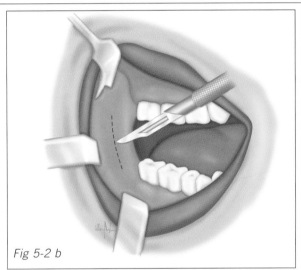

Fig 5-2 b

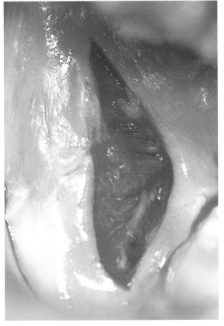

Fig 5-2 c

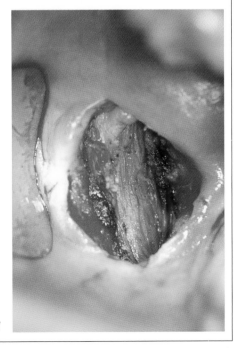

Fig 5-2 d

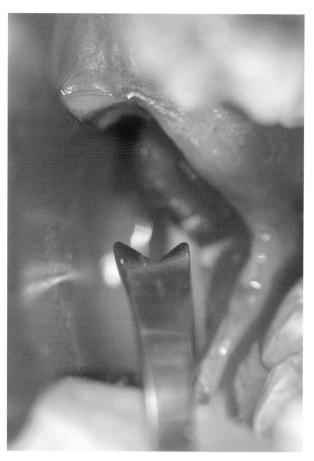

Fig 5-3 A bifurcated periosteal elevator is of great help in peeling off the tendious insertions of the temporalis muscle.

When performing the incision, palpation of the anterior border of the ascending ramus is essential to avoid deviations to the lingual side that might cause trauma to the lingual or the inferior alveolar nerves.

Dissection should then proceed with a bifurcated periosteal elevator, peeling up from the bone both periosteum and tendinous insertions from the temporalis muscle (Fig 5-3). Often we find it necessary to use a scalpel to release some deep tendinous insertions from the bone (Fig 5-4). Should this be the case, peeling off these fibrous remnants from the graft is recommended.

It is of utmost importance to find the lower limit of the sigmoid notch, since it will pinpoint the lower end of our graft.

Once de-globing of the CP is achieved, the surrounding soft tissues should be protected with retractors (Langenbeck, Minnesota, Obwegeser). A horizontal osteotomy is then undertaken. For this purpose, we favour the use of a reciprocating saw. Lindemann or fissure burs are good alternatives (Fig 5-5 a-c). Rotary instruments, however, are more prone to get stuck in the surrounding soft tissues, with a greater risk of neural or vascular damage.

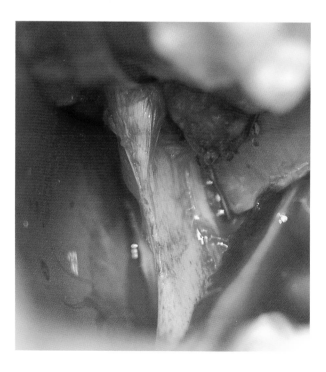

Fig 5-4 Access to the CP is easier through the lingual side, and finding the inferior limit of the sigmoid notch should be done from this side.

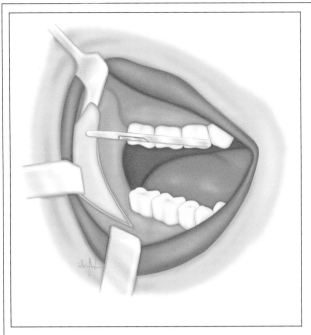

Fig 5-5 a

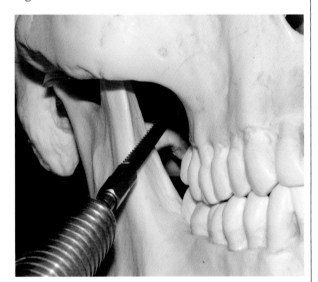

Fig 5-5 b

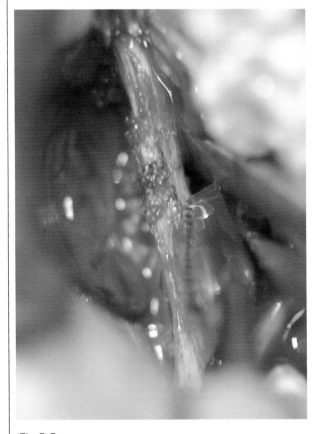

Fig 5-5 c

Fig 5-5 d

Fig 5-5 (a-c) A reciprocating saw is the easiest, fastest and least traumatic tool to perform the osteotomy. Note how a bone clamp is holding the CP during osteotomy to avoid dislodgement into the temporalis fossa.

As a general precaution we recommend using a bone clamp to hold the CP while carrying out the osteotomy (Fig 5-6). This avoids superior displacement and eventual disappearance of the graft if some muscular insertions are still attached after freeing of the graft.

After graft harvesting careful inspection will detect bleeding points that should be identified and cauterised.

By lengthening the incision downwards by a few millimetres the whole anterior aspect of the ascending ramus will be exposed and thus further grafts can be harvested from this area.

Closing of the incision can be done with a running 4/0 resorbable suture, being careful to include muscle and mucosa within the sutured flaps (Fig 5-7).

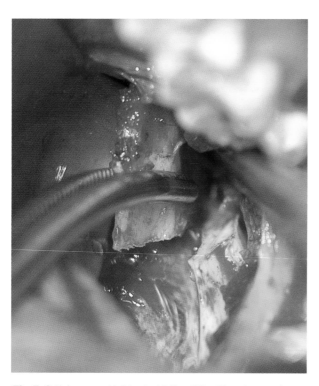

Fig 5-6 It is essential to hold the CP with a bone clamp before completely releasing muscle and tendinous insertions to avoid displacement into the temporalis fossa.

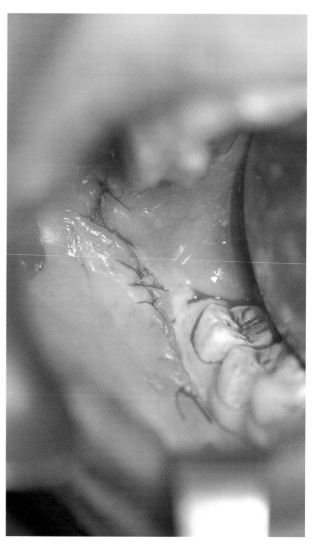

Fig 5-7 A running 4/0 suture should re-approach muscle and mucosa.

Clinical Applications

Youmans[1] was the first to publish the use of this graft for small defects in the mandible. More recently[2,3] it has been proposed for reconstructions of the floor of the orbit in blow-out fractures, and as an onlay graft for correction of paranasal deficiencies.[4]

In oral implantology and preprosthetic surgery it has a role as an onlay graft in different clinical situations where a limited amount of a rather cortical bone is needed.

Obviously it is not a first choice for big 3-D defects due to its flat shape, even though it can be milled and thus used to fill medium-sized cavities.

Complications

Reported complications of the technique include haemorrhage, swelling at the donor site and variable degrees of swelling.[4,5] Disinsertion of some tendinous fibres of the temporalis muscle does not seem to affect chewing function after a few days.

To reduce inflammation we recommend injection of corticosteroids into the bulk of the temporalis muscle once the grafting procedure is finished. Variable degrees of limitation in mouth-opening can be anticipated with this technique but will soon improve.

As pointed out earlier, it is of utmost importance to clamp the CP and completely release the tendinous insertions before completing the osteotomy to avoid displacement of the graft into the temporalis fossa due to the muscle pull.

The most serious complication with this procedure would be severing of the inferior alveolar bundle. This can be easily avoided by careful subperiosteal dissection and using retractors to protect the surrounding soft tissues.

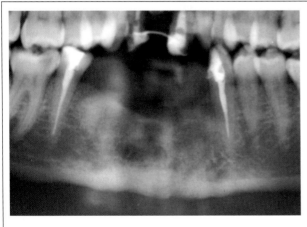

Fig 5-8 a

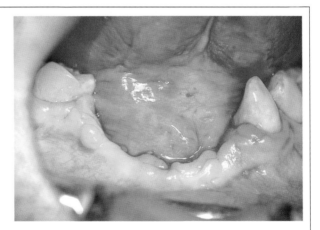

Fig 5-8 b

Fig 5-8 (a, b) Vertical and AP defect of the anterior mandible secondary to trauma. Reconstruction is planned with coronoid process and trephined bone from the symphisys.

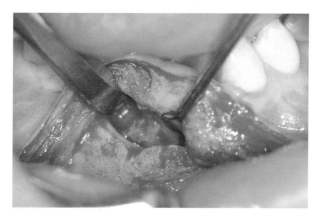

Fig 5-8 (c) Left CP with fibrous remnants already peeled off. Careful evaluation of the defect and available material is critical to achieve satisfactory reconstructions.

Fig 5-8 (d) A vestibular incision gives access to the defective site. When performing de-globing of the area, it is of utmost importance to preserve integrity of the periosteal layer.

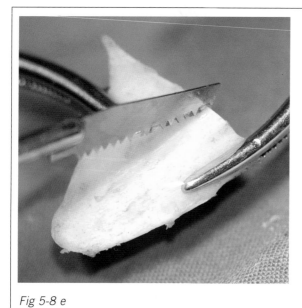

Fig 5-8 e

Fig 5-8 f

Fig 5-8 (e, f) The thin cut of a reciprocating saw or a disc is needed to cut the graft, thus minimising loss of bone.

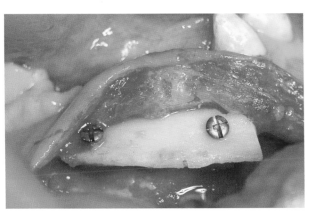

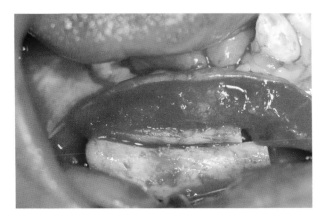

Fig 5-8 (g) Two screws are used to stabilise one of the bone pieces in a 'tent' fashion.

Fig 5-8 (h) One more piece creates the vestibular 'wall'.

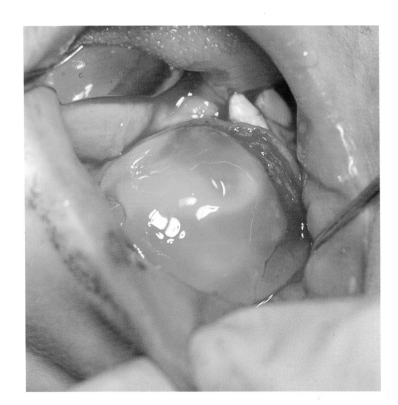

Fig 5-8 (i) Trephined bone from the chin mixed with PRP is placed under this 'box'.

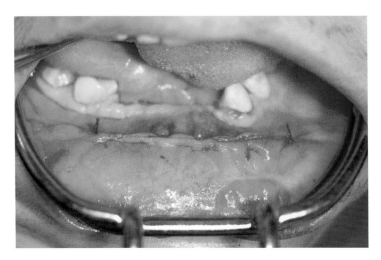

Fig 5-8 (j) A watertight closure in two layers (periosteum-muscle and mucosa respectively) is achieved in order to preserve isolation of the grafts.

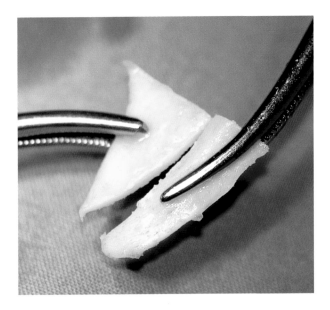

Fig 5-9 (a) A right coronoid process is divided into two to reconstruct, in a veneer fashion, a double vestibular defect at the anterior maxilla.

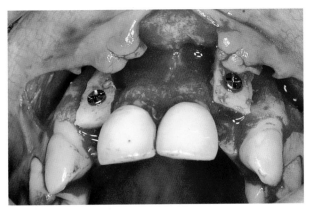

Fig 5-9 (b) Split pieces of the graft held in place with two screws.

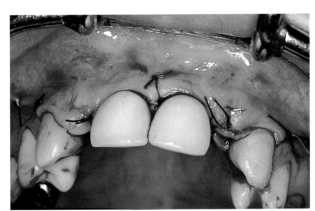

Fig 5-9 (c) Primary closure.

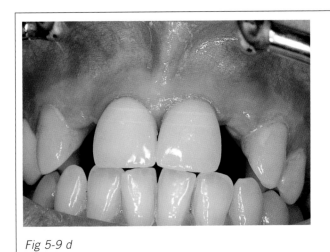

Fig 5-9 d

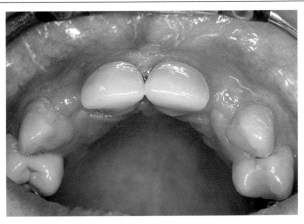

Fig 5-9 e

Fig 5-9 (d, e) Clinical aspect two months after first surgery.

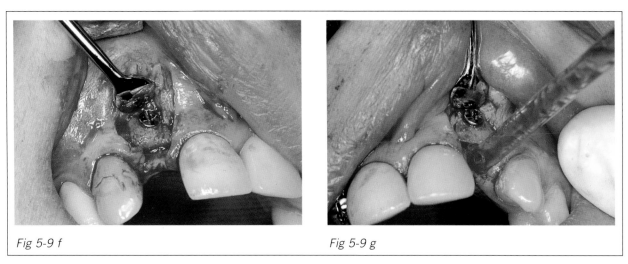

Fig 5-9 f

Fig 5-9 g

Fig 5-9 (f, g) Flap design should preserve the papillae.

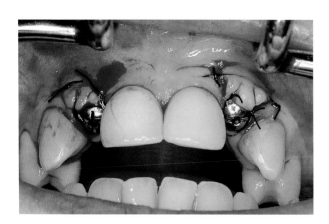

Fig 5-9 (h) Two fixtures placed in a one-stage fashion are positioned after screw removal.

117

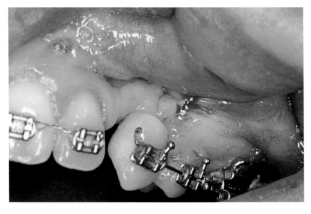

Fig 5-10 (a) Alveolar cleft. Orthodontic treatment to open space is followed by reconstruction of the defect.

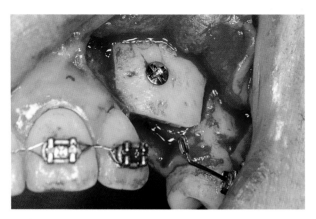

Fig 5-10 (b) A graft from the CP is harvested and fixed with one screw that travels obliquely to engage the palatal vault. The rest of the graft is milled and placed under the main block.

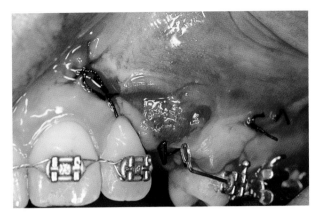

Fig 5-10 (c) Primary closure.

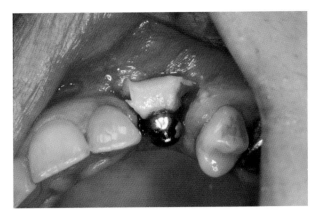

Fig 5-10 (d) Re-entry three months later, placing the fixture in one stage.

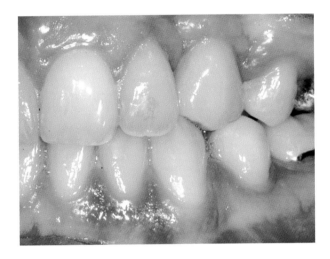

Fig 5-10 (e) Final result.

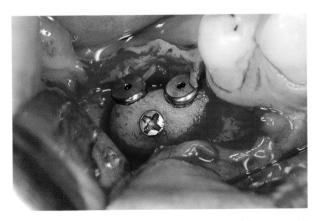

Fig 5-11 (a) Vestibular augmentation with coronoid graft and simultaneous placement of fixtures at the posterior mandible.

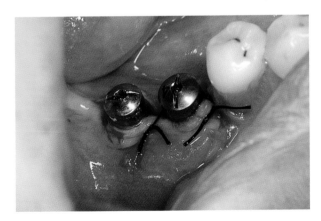

Fig 5-11 (b) Abutment connection

References

1 Youmans R, Russell E. The coronoid process: A new donor source for autogenous bone grafts. Oral Surg Oral Med Oral Pathol 1969;27:422.

2 Mintz SM, Ettinger A, Schamakel T, Gleason MJ. Contralateral coronoid process bone grafts for orbital floor reconstruction: An anatomic and clinical study. J Oral Maxillofac Surg 1998;56:1140-1144.

3 Hönig JF. The coronoid proceOss as a new donor source for autogenous bone grafts for reconstructing orbital and midface defects. Bull Group Int Rech Sci Stomatol Odontol 1996;39:49-55.

4 Choung PH, Kim SG. The coronoid process for paranasal augmentation in the correction of midface concavity. Oral Surg Oral Med Oral Pathol 2001;91:28-33.

5 Johnson JV. Discussion of contralateral coronoid process bone grafts for orbital floor reconstruction: An anatomic and clinical study. J. Oral Maxillofac Surg 1998;56:1144-5.

6 Maxillary Tuberosity

Surgical Anatomy

The maxillary tuberosity (MT) constitutes the posterior limit of the upper maxilla and is located distally to the upper second molar (Fig 6-1). It has a round and thick aspect, with its upper part being smooth and constituting the anterior wall of the pterigomaxillary space. Both the upper maxillary nerve and the sphenopalatine artery wander through this space. The lower part of the tuberosity articulates with the palatine bone.

The anterior aspect of the tuberosity shares its limits with the maxillary sinus, and when considering the harvest of bone from this area care should be taken not to violate the integrity of the sinus in order to avoid a secondary oroantral fistula. The best way to avoid this complication is by a thorough radiological exam either by panoramic X-ray or CT scan.

An interesting fact regarding this area is the frequent finding of impacted upper third molars. If this is the case they might reduce the amount of available bone. On the other hand, when they need removal the same approach will suffice and allow harvesting of bone chips from the area.

Regarding bone quality, the MT is usually composed of cancellous soft bone (type 3 and 4 according to Lekholm's classification), surrounded by a thin cortical layer. The origin of this bone is membranous.

121

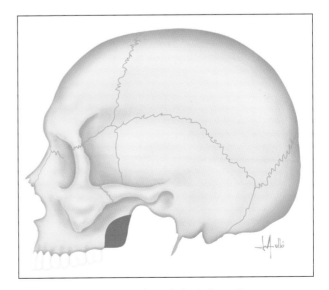

Fig 6-1 Anatomic location of the tuberosity.

Surgical Technique

Local infiltrative anaesthesia at both the vestibule and the palatal area is sufficient to harvest bone from the MT.

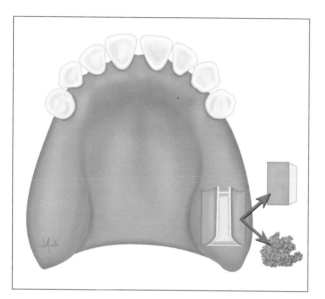

Fig 6-2 When the third molar is absent, an 'H' type incision allows easy access. Then either a block or a small amount of soft bone can be harvested.

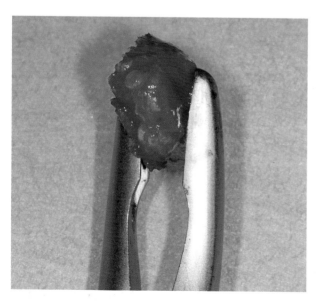

Fig 6-3 A bone rongeur is helpful to bite bone 'chunks'.

Approach to the area is the same as when removing an upper third molar. A longitudinal incision on the crest is followed by a relieving vestibular incision medially. If the third molar is absent, an 'H' type incision allows easy access (Fig 6-2). Careful subperiosteal dissection allows visualisation of the area.

If a third molar is to be removed at the same procedure, it is advisable to perform the ostectomy with a chisel or a rongeur, avoiding the use of burs. A small bone block will thus be obtained while gaining access to the molar. Once it has been removed a rongeur will assist in nibbling the area to get additional bone chips (Fig 6-3).

If the molar is absent it is possible to harvest a rather larger block from the area that can be used as such or milled to fill a space (Fig 6-4).

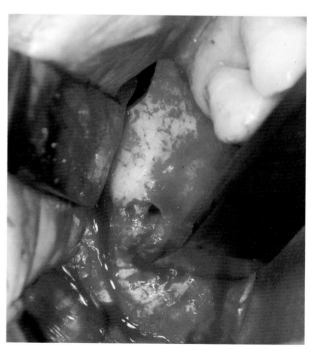

Fig 6-4 When the third molar is absent, it is easy to harvest a block with the aid of a chisel. Rotary instruments should not be used in this area to avoid tearing soft tissues.

If a bur is used to perform the ostectomy it is essential to use a bone filter to avoid losing the mobilised bone shavings.

Occasionally we might enter the maxillary sinus. To avoid the possibility of an oro-antral fistula, we recommend the use of the buccal fat pad. A small stab incision in the periosteum at this level will suffice to provoke herniation of the pad. This manoeuvre should always be carried out after completion of the harvesting procedure.

This area is also an excellent source of connective tissue grafts. The palatal flap developed to gain access to the area is usually thick enough and consists of a good connective tissue stock.

Suturing of the flaps is done with resorbable 4/0 sutures.

Clinical Applications

Harvested bone from the tuberosity is usually scarce, which means that in most instances it will be used to solve small vertical or horizontal defects,[1] filling of small cavities, exposure of fixture threads and filling of post-extraction sockets. It has been also proposed as filling material for sinus lift procedures (Fig 6-5 a-j, Fig 6-6 a-d).[2,3]

When harvested as a block it can be stabilised with a screw or impacted at the recipient zone (Fig 6-7 a-l).

Complications

Oroantral communication is a rare complication of this harvesting procedure. Should an oro-antral communication occur after harvesting it is advisable to seal it with a buccal fat pad flap. This flap is right behind the tuberosity.[4]

Minimal morbitity can be expected when using the tuberosity as a donor site. In our experience, limiting the relieving incision contributes to a reduction in postoperative oedema and pain.

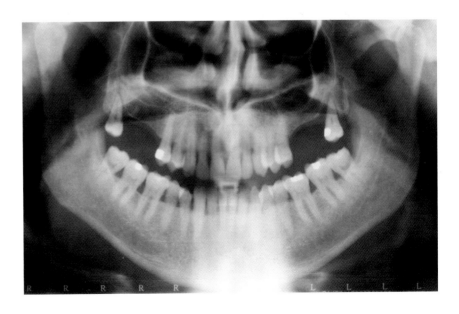

Fig 6-5 (a) Patient presenting with bilateral posterior edentulism in the maxilla. A bilateral sinus lift was planned and both tuberosities were selected as donor sites. Upper third molar removal was also planned.

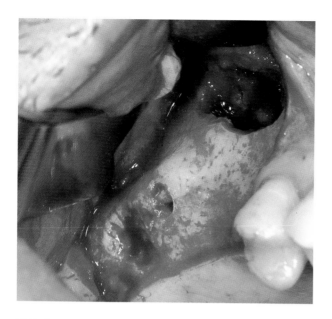

Fig 6-5 (b) Close-up view of the right side. Third molar removal is followed by access to the sinus and preparation of the cavity.

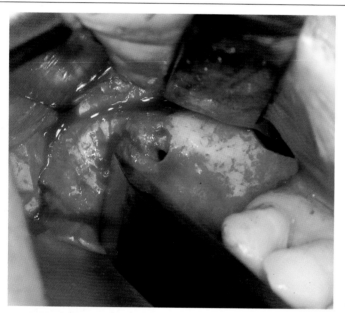

Fig 6-5 (c, d) A chisel is used to harvest a block from the tuberosity.

Fig 6-5 c

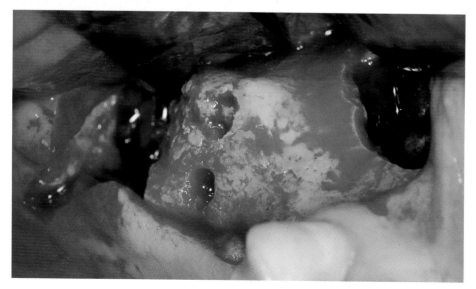

Fig 6-5 d

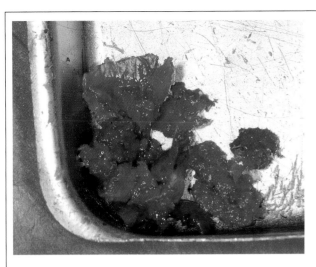

Fig 6-5 e

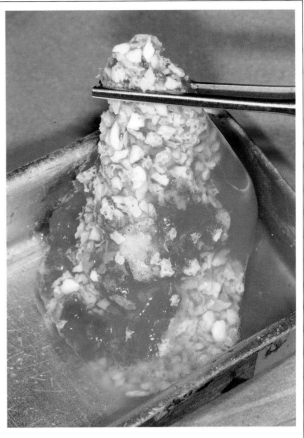

Fig 6-5 (e, f) Harvested bone is milled and mixed with anorganic bone matrix and PRP.

Fig 6-5 f

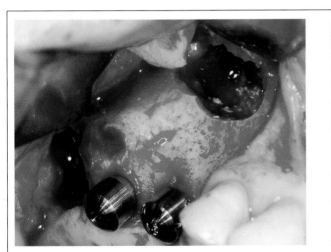

Fig 6-5 g

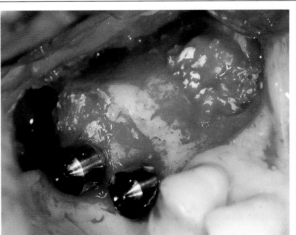

Fig 6-5 h

Fig 6-5 (g, h) The sinus cavity is filled with the graft and two fixtures are placed simultaneously, as the residual bone guaranteed their stability. Note how the graft has also been used to reconstruct the donor site.

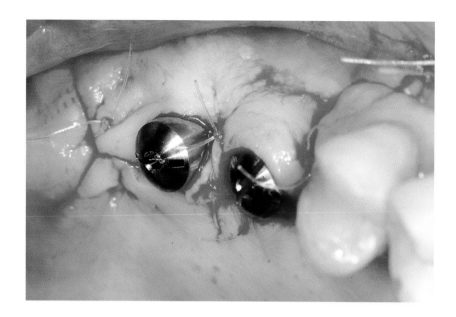

Fig 6-5 (i) Immediate abutment connection and suturing with 5/0 monofilament.

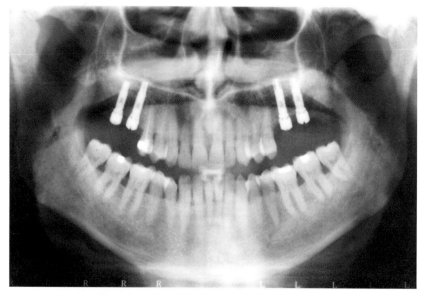

126

Fig 6-5 (j) The same procedure carried out on the opposite side. Panoramix X-ray showing the result. This case illustrates how a single surgical procedure and a single surgical site may, at times, solve moderate reconstructive problems.

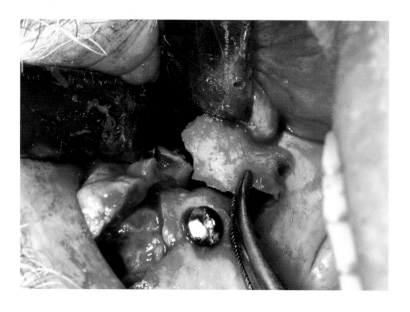

Fig 6-6 (a) Bone block harvested from left tuberosity to cover a crestal defect after implant failure.

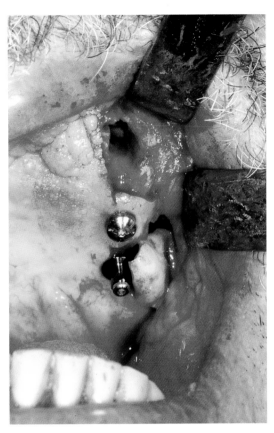

Fig 6-6 (b) The defect in the bicuspid area is curetted.

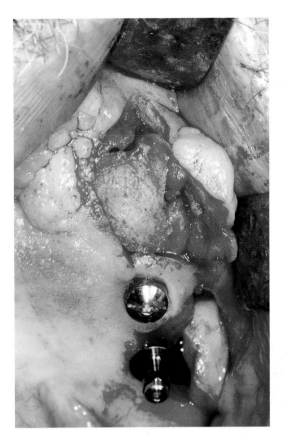

Fig 6-6 (c) Bone graft adapted to cover the area.

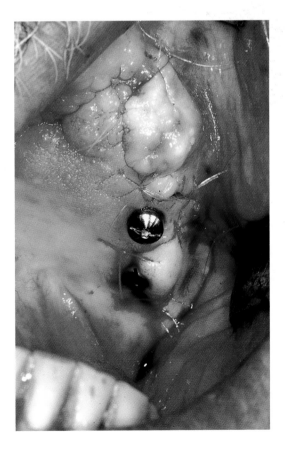

Fig 6-6 (d) Soft tissue is trimmed to protect the reconstruction. In this case the bone graft acts as a biologic membrane to isolate the cavity and to preserve it from soft tissue in-growth.

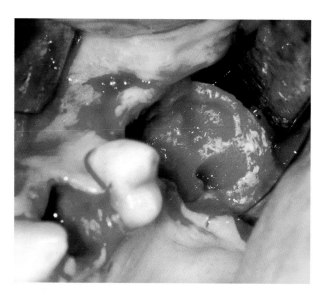

Fig 6-7 (a) Panoramic X-ray showing severe periodontal compromise at the upper left second and third molar. Note also loss of support mesially to the upper right second molar. There is also a fracture at the upper left first bicuspid.

Fig 6-7 (b) Tri-dimensional bone defect after removal of the left molars. Note the tuberosity behind the alveolus of the third molar.

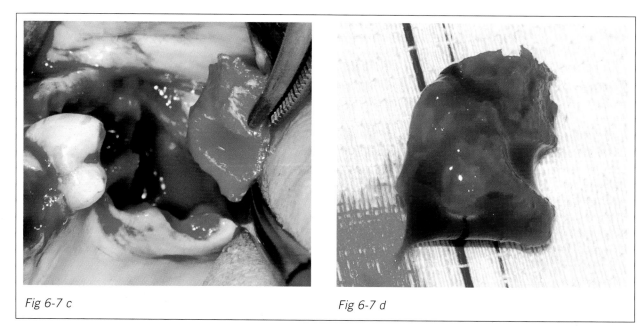

Fig 6-7 c

Fig 6-7 d

Fig 6-7 (c, d) A bone block is removed from the tuberosity with the aid of a chisel.

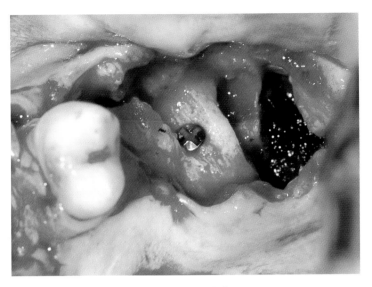

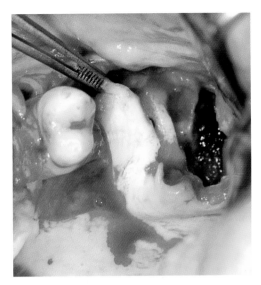

Fig 6-7 (e) The block is fixed in the defect.

Fig 6-7 (f) A split flap from the palate is used to aid in coverage of the reconstruction.

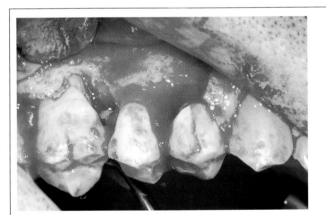

Fig 6-7 g

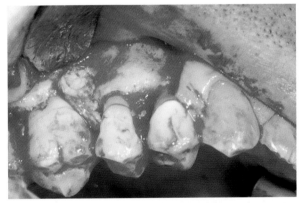

Fig 6-7 h

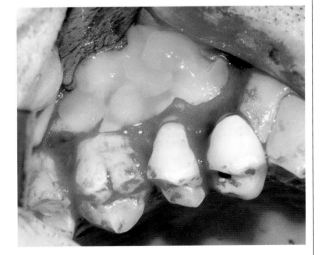

Fig 6-7 i

Fig 6-7 (g-i) Extra bone chips from the same site are used together with PRP to reconstruct the contralateral defect.

Fig 6-7 (j) Re-entry four months later, allowing screw removal.

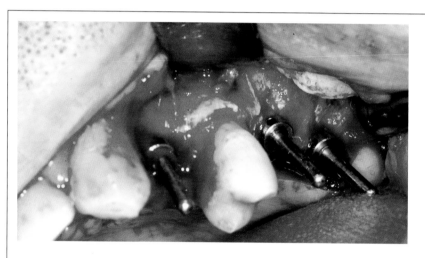

Fig 6-7 k

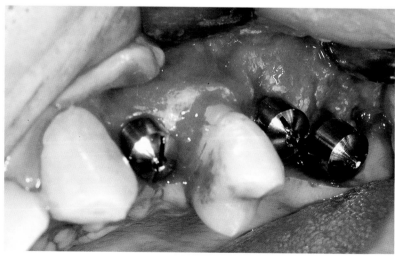

Fig 6-7 l

Fig 6-7 (k, l) Fixture installation in completely regenerated bone. This case illustrates again that often the best donor sites are immediately adjacent to the defect.

References

1 Moenning JE, Graham LL. Elimination of mandibular labial undercut with autogenous bone graft from a maxillary tuberosity. J Prosthetic Dentistry 1986;56:211-214.

2 Raghoebar GM, Brouwer TJ, Reintsema H, Oort V. Augmentation of the maxillary sinus floor with autogenous bone for the placement of endosseous implants: A preliminary report. J Oral Maxillofac Surg 1993;51:1198-1203.

3 Raghoebar GM, Timmenga NM, Reintsema H, et al. Maxillary bone grafting for insertion of endosseous implants: Results after 12-24 months. Clin Oral Impl Res 2001;12:279-286

4 Martin-Granizo R, Naval L, Costas A, et al. Use of buccal fat pad to repair intraoral defects: Review of 30 cases. Br J Oral Maxillofac Surg 1997;35:81-84.

131

Sinus Wall

Surgical Anatomy

The anterior sinus wall (SW) constitutes the anterior limit of the maxillary sinus and is the usual access area to perform a sinus lift procedure. It is made of a thin cortical bone, which can be easily cut with the aid of a fissure bur or even with piezoelectric instruments. The infraorbital foramen is the upper limit for SW harvesting (Fig 7-1).

The infraorbital nerve is the key landmark to bear in mind and respect when approaching this area. It is placed 5-7mm under the inferior limit of the orbit.[1]

The posterior teeth also have an intimate relationship with the maxillary sinus.[2]

Another important anatomical fact regarding the sinus is the frequent presence of bony septa originating in the floor of the sinus.[3] Dissection of the membrane at this level may be especially difficult.

The sinus membrane, also known as Schneiderian membrane, acts as a defence mechanisms, trapping particles in the mucus and conducting them to the ostium.[4]

Normal sinus volume in adults varies between 4 and 35cc (mean 15cc). Age and tooth loss, together with osteoclastic activity of the mem-

133

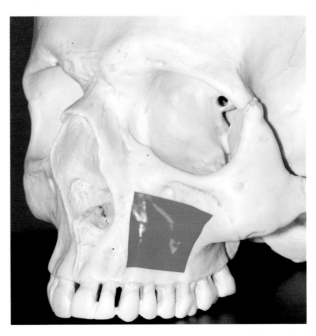

Fig 7-1 Limits of the anterior wall of the maxilla. Infra-orbital nerve, zygomatic buttress, alveolar process, and piriform or paranasal buttress.

brane, seem to be responsible for the progressive pneumatisation of the sinus.[5]

Surgical Procedure

Anaesthesia

Infraorbital nerve block plus infiltrative anaesthesia will suffice to harvest grafts from these areas. Only additional complex procedures would justify the use of sedation or general anaesthesia.

Access

In cases of simultaneous sinus lift procedures and/or placement of implants, the incision should be placed at the alveolar crest. When the graft is to be used at a different place within the oral cavity, a vestibular incision can be carried out at least 2mm over the mucogingival junction to allow easy suturing after the procedure.

Periosteal elevation follows in an upward fashion to reach the level of the infraorbital nerve. This will be the upper security limit (Fig 7-2a).

Laterally subperiosteal dissection should proceed over the zygomatic buttress. When done as a pure harvesting procedure, the sinus membrane does not have to be lifted from the sinus floor. Design of the window is followed by its removal and resuturing of the mucoperiosteal flap in place (Fig 7-2 b, c).

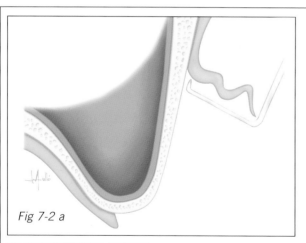

Fig 7-2 a

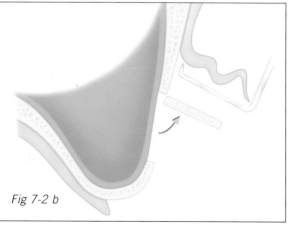

Fig 7-2 b

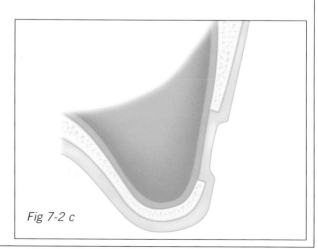

Fig 7-2 c

Fig 7-2 (a-c) Dissection proceeds as in a conventional sinus lift. The window is removed and sinus mucosa and periosteum remain together after the procedure. Compression over the infraorbital nerve should be avoided.

Harvesting procedure

To harvest bone from the SW we recommend either fissure burs or ultrasounds.

The former has the advantage of speed but is more technically sensitive (Fig 7-3 a, b). Ultrasounds are safer regarding preservation of the sinus mucosa but much slower (Fig 7-4). A midway solution is using fissure diamond burs.

Once designed, the bony window is lifted just like in any sinus-lift procedure.[6-8]

Running 4/0 resorbable sutures can be used for closing.

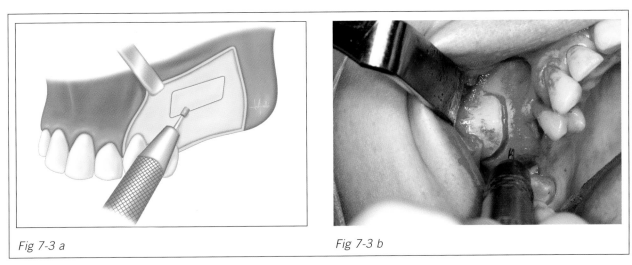

Fig 7-3 a   Fig 7-3 b

Fig 7-3 (a, b) Graft harvest with fissure bur. Easy, fast but technically sensitive due to the risk of severing the membrane.

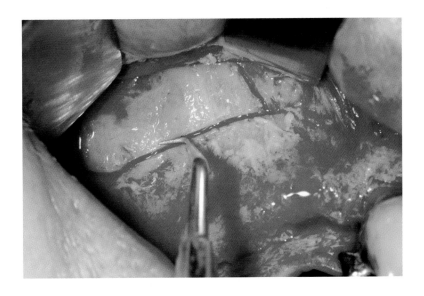

Fig 7-4 Piezoelectric osteotomy is safer but slower.

Clinical Applications

The use of the anterior maxillary wall as a graft has been advocated to reconstruct the orbital floor in blow-out fractures.[9-12]

SW is an autologous rigid membrane that has the same applications as any membrane with such characteristics (for instance, reconstruc-

tion of alveolar walls, protection of particulated or cancellous bone).[13]

In three-wall defects it may be useful to bridge the defect and avoid collapse of the muco-periosteal layer (Fig 7-5).[14]

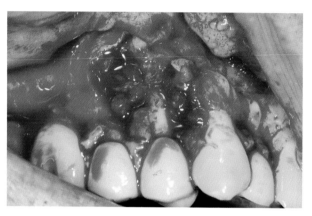

Fig 7-5 (a) Granulomatous endo-perio process involving two upper bicuspids.

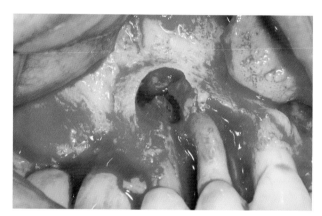

Fig 7-5 (b) Thorough curettage yields a moderate three-wall defect. Root amputation is decided upon, considering the poor prognosis of both teeth.

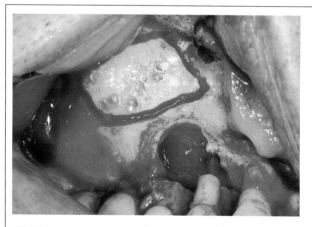

Fig 7-5 c

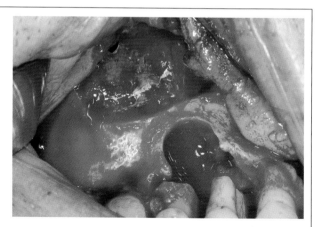

Fig 7-5 d

Fig 7-5 (c, d) Immediate reconstruction of the defect is decided upon. The filler will be anorganic bone matrix with PRP. A bone graft from the anterior maxillary wall is harvested, both to protect the reconstruction and to help in regeneration of the lost vestibular wall.

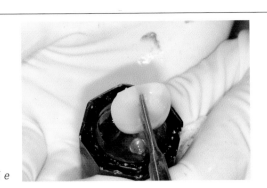

Fig 7-5 e

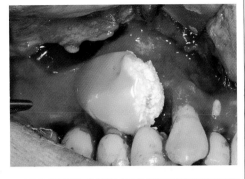

Fig 7-5 f

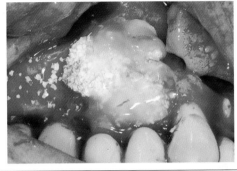

Fig 7-5 (e-g) PRP helps in managing the particulated matrix.

Fig 7-5 g

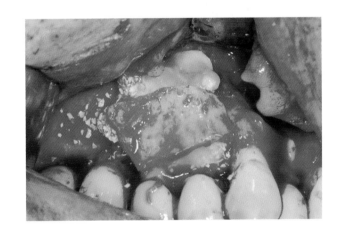

Fig 7-5 (h) The bony membrane is applied covering the lateral defect.

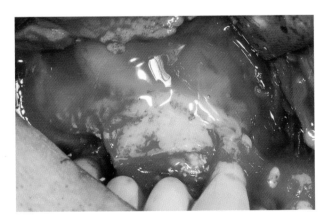

Fig 7-5 (i) PRP aids in primary stabilisation of the bone plate.

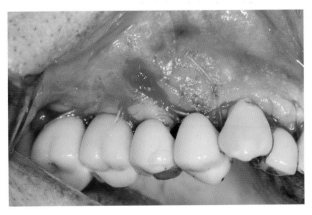

Fig 7-5 (j) Meticulous suturing of the flaps is completed after relieving the vestibular flap with periosteal incisions.

The use of PRP in combination with different biomaterials has been proposed by different authors.[15,16] In these instances the anterior wall may be used to protect the reconstruction and avoid fibrous in-growth (Fig 7-6 and 7-7).

Different studies have shown how particulated bone collected with a bone filter while preparing implant sockets, suffices to cover exposed threads in selected cases.[17] SW can be used for the same purpose as a conventional membrane without additional costs for the patient.

The same principles would apply to reconstruct vestibular walls following extraction of periodontally compromised teeth as a means of preparing future sites for the fixtures.[18-20]

In summary, these areas are especially useful when the defective area is in the vicinity or when a thin lamina of bone is needed. Otherwise, we recommend either the mandible or the tuberosity for harvesting.

Complications

Neural: Excessive traction or compression of the infraorbital nerve can produce transient or prolonged anaesthesia of the cheek.

Sinusal: Perforation of the sinus membrane will have no ill effects in the majority of cases. However, in cases with a concomitant sinus lift procedure, membrane preservation is essential.

Trismus: Stripping of the masseter muscle from the zygomatic buttress may produce transient masticatory dysfunction. When fibres are transsected it is advisable to inject corticosteroids locally.

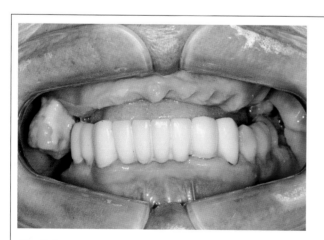

Fig 7-6 a

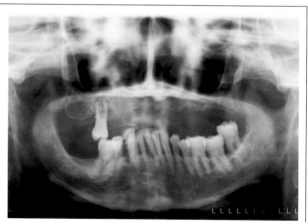

Fig 7-6 b

Fig 7-6 (a, b) Bilateral atrophic maxilla. The plan is to perform a bilateral sinus lift procedure, grafting with cancellous bone from the tibia, and simultaneous placement of implants. Note the presence of an upper second molar with a severe periodontal defect.

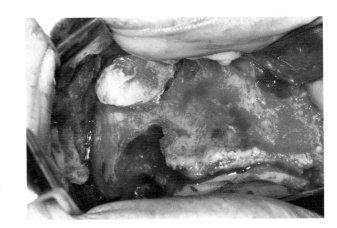

Fig 7-6 (c) On the right side the access window to perform the sinus lift is removed. Note a three-wall crestal defect after removal of the molar and thorough curettage.

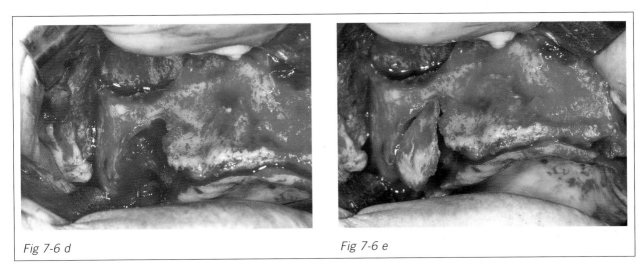

Fig 7-6 d   Fig 7-6 e

Fig 7-6 (d, e) The anterior wall of the maxillary sinus has been removed. Note preservation of membrane integrity to allow reconstruction. The 'bone membrane' is adapted to the vestibular wall defect.

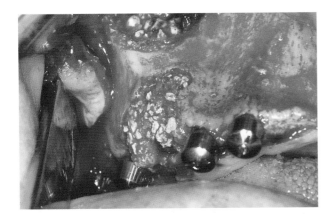

Fig 7-6 (f) Grafted material from the tibia is mixed with bovine inorganic matrix and used to fill both the sinus and the crestal defect. Implants have already been placed.

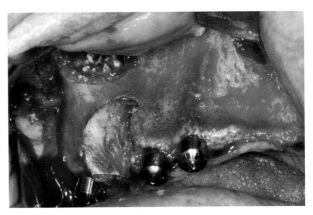

Fig 7-6 (g) The bone plate is adapted and positioned in place.

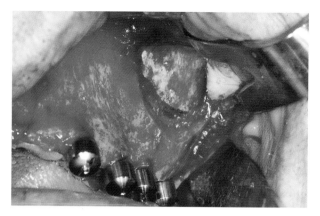

Fig 7-6 (h) Sinus lift is completed at the contralateral side.

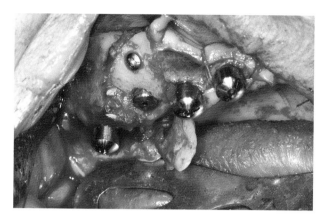

Fig 7-6 (i) After fixation of the bone plate with a screw, a last implant is positioned at this level. This implant is stabilised apically and sufficient compression of the particulated bone provides stability.

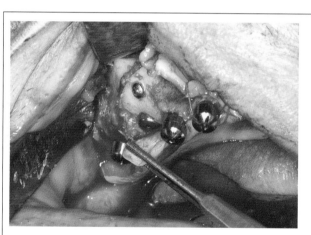

Fig 7-6 j

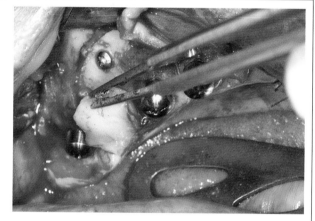

Fig 7-6 k

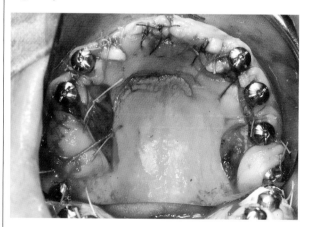

Fig 7-6 l

Fig 7-6 (j-l) To cover the reconstruction, a palatal split-thickness pedicled flap is developed. It is important to perform adequate soft tissue coverage with keratinised mucosa.

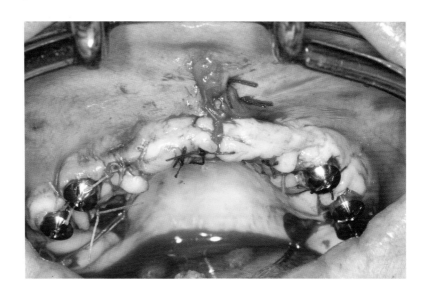

Fig 7-6 (m) Primary closure after abutment connection of all except one of the fixtures; the one located at the crestal reconstruction site.

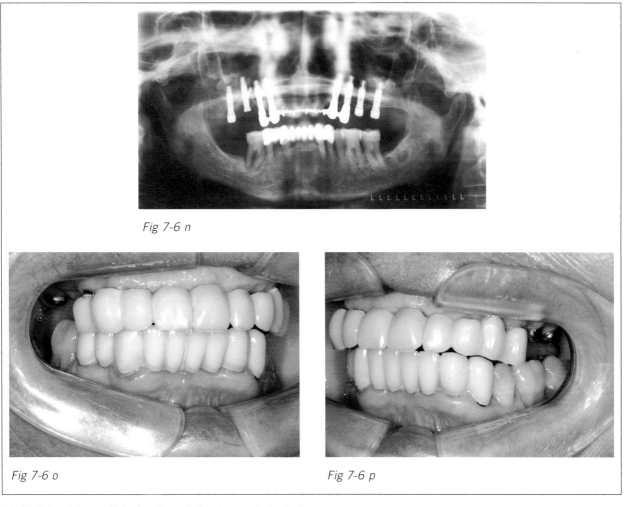

Fig 7-6 n

Fig 7-6 o

Fig 7-6 p

Fig 7-6 (n-p) Immediate loading of the four anterior fixtures.

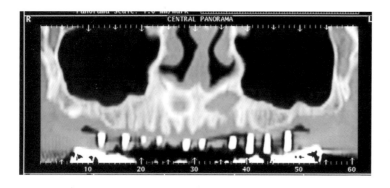

Fig 7-7 (a) A bilateral sinus lift was planned in a patient with a history of chronic sinusitis. The sinus membrane was disrupted bilaterally during elevation.

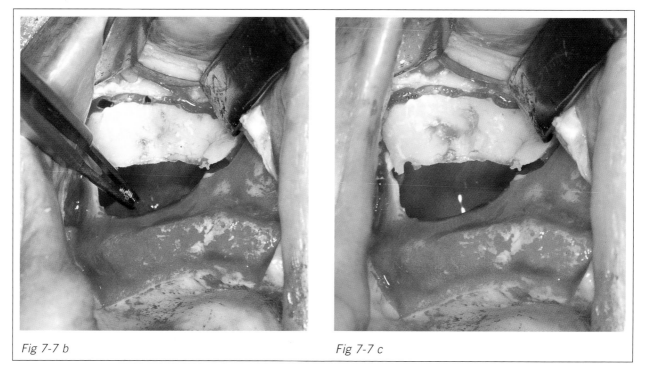

Fig 7-7 b   *Fig 7-7 c*

Fig 7-7 (b, c) A bone graft from the anterior maxillary sinus wall was harvested to be used as the roof for the new reconstruction.

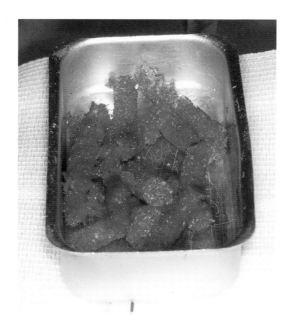

Fig 7-7 (d) The filling material was harvested from the tibia as previously planned.

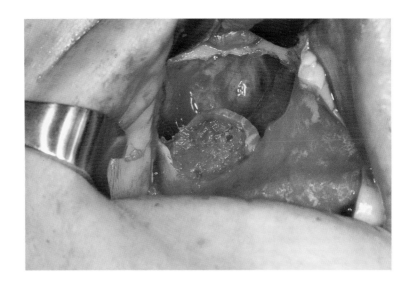

Fig 7-7 (e) 'Box' reconstruction within the sinus. Note how cancellous bone from the tibia is covered by the graft obtained from the anterior sinus wall, thus preventing dislodgement of particles into the sinus.

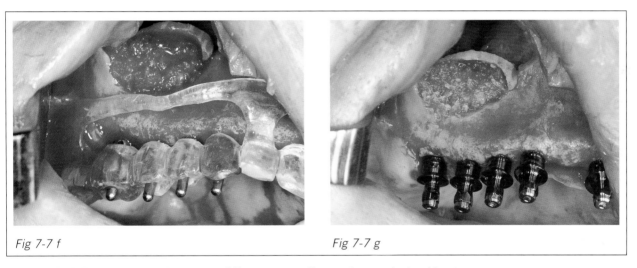

Fig 7-7 f   *Fig 7-7 g*

Fig 7-7 (f, g) Simultaneous placement of fixtures according to the surgical guide.

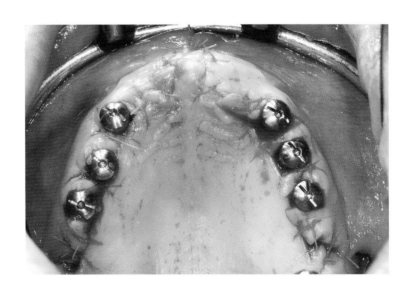

Fig 7-7 (h) Abutment connection was followed by tailoring of the flaps. This facilitates both papilla regeneration between fixtures and seal of the reconstructed area.

References

1   Figun ME, Garino RR. Anatomía Odontológica funcional y aplicada. Buenos Aires: El Ateneo, 1988.

2   Jensen OT. The Sinus Bone Graft. Illinois: Quintessence, 1999.

3   Ulm CW, Solar P, Kremmair G, et al. Incidence and surgical management of septa in sinus-lift procedures. Int J Oral Maxillofac Implants 1995;10:462.

4   Chavanaz M. Maxillary Sinus: Anatomy, physiology, surgery and bone grafting related to implantology: Eleven years of surgical experience (1979-1990). J Oral Implantol 1990;16:199.

5   Ulm CW, Solar P, Gsellmann B, et al. The edentulous maxillary alveolar process in the region of the maxillary sinus: A study of physical dimensions. Int J Oral Maxillofac Surg 1995;24:279.

6   Manisch O, Lozada JL, Holmes RE, et al. Maxillary sinus augmentation prior to placement of endosseous implants: A histomorphometric analysis. Int J Oral Maxillofac Implants 1999;14:329.

7   Moy PK, Lundgren S, Holmes RE. Maxillary sinus augmentation: Histomorphometric analysis of graft materials for maxillary sinus floor augmentation. J Oral Maxillofac Surg 1993;51:857.

8   Maiorana C, Redemagni M, Rabagliati M, Salina S. Treatment of maxillary ridge resorption by sinus augmentation with iliac cancellous bone, anorganic bovine bone and endosseous implants. Int J Oral Maxillofac Implants 2000;15:873.

9   Pearl RM, Defiebre B Jr. The versatile anterior maxillary wall bone graft. Ann Plast Surg 1981;7:191.

10 Kaye BL. Orbital floor repair with antral wall bone grafts. Plast Reconstr Surg. 1996; 37:62.

11 Roncevic R, Stajcic Z. Surgical treatment of posttraumatic enophtalmos: A study of 72 patients. Ann Plast Surg 1994;32:288.

12 Hayasaka S, Aikawa Y, Wada M, et al. Transconjuntival and transantral approaches are combined with antral wall bone graft to repair orbital floor blow-out fractures. Ophtalmologica 1994; 208:284.

13 Mish M. Comparison of intraoral donor sites for onlay grafting prior to implant placement. Int J Oral Maxillofac Implants 1997;12:767.

14 Baladron J, Junquera LM, Clavero A, Clavero B. Injertos óseos en cirugía implantológica: Técnicas quirúrgicas en el maxilar y la mandíbula. Rev Esp Cirug Oral y Maxilofac. 2001; 23:144.

15 Dahlin C, Lekholm U, Becker W. Treatment of fenestration and dehiscence bone defects around oral implants using the guided tissue regeneration technique: a prospective multicenter study. Int J Oral Maxillofac Implants 1995;10:312.

16 Zitzmam NV, Naef R, Schärer P. Resorbable versus nonresorbable membrane in combination with Bio-Oss for guided bone regeneration. Int J Oral Maxillofac Implants 1997;12:844.

17 Widmark G, Ivanoff CJ Augmentation of exposed implant threads with autogenous bone chips: Prospective clinical study. Clin Impl Dent Relat Res 2000;2:178.

18 Smukler H, Landi L, Setayesh R. Histomorphometric evaluation of extraction sockets and deficient alveolar ridges treated with allograft and barrier membrane: A pilot study. Int J Oral Maxillofac Implants1999;14:407.

19 Henry PJ, Tan A, Leavy J, et al. Tissue regeneration in bony defects adjacent to immediately loaded titanium implants placed into extraction sockets: A study in dogs. Int J Oral Maxillofac Implants 1997;12:758.

20 Peni de Carvalho, Wovascancelos L, Pi J. Influence of bed preparation on the incorporation of autogenous bone grafts: A study in dogs. Int J Oral Maxillofac Implants 2000; 15:565.

8 Zygomatic Buttress

Surgical Anatomy

The zygomatic buttress (ZB) is formed by the junction of the zygomatic process of the maxilla and the maxillary process of the malar bone. The quality and density of bone in this location compensates for the paucity of material that can be harvested. Its location facilitates the procedure, especially for minor defects in the maxillary region.

The zygomatic buttress is responsible for supporting the forces applied to the maxilla via the mandible and its attached masticatory muscles. The zygomatic buttress forms the anterolateral limit of the sinus, and in certain sinus lift procedures the access window is designed on it.[1]

One of the key anatomic points to bear in mind when harvesting bone from either the ZB or the SW is the infraorbital foramen which gives exit to the infraorbital nerve. Flap retractors should be positioned away from this area to avoid stretching or compressing the nerve, thus provoking paraesthesia in the region.

CT scan studies of the area will allow determination of the amount of bone present and its density.[2]

Surgical Procedure

Anaesthesia

Infraorbital nerve block plus infiltrative anaesthesia will suffice to harvest grafts from these areas. Only additional complex procedures would justify the use of sedation or general anaesthesia.

Access

In cases of simultaneous sinus lift procedures and/or placement of implants, incisions should be placed at the alveolar crest. When harvesting the graft for a distant application within the oral cavity, a vestibular incision can be made at least 2mm over the mucogingival junction to allow easy suturing after the procedure (Fig 8-1).

Periosteal elevation follows in an upward fashion to reach the level of the infraorbital nerve. This will be the upper security limit.

Laterally, subperiosteal dissection should proceed over the zygomatic buttress. At this point we will find insertions of the masseter muscle that have to be carefully stripped off the bone.

Harvesting procedure

At this point a distinction should be made between ZB and SW. The former, as stated pre-

viously, is solid, thick cortical bone. Harvesting procedures include:

- Trephine: obtaining bone cores (Fig 8-2).
- Bone scrapper: Obtaining particles of cortical bone (Fig 8-3a, b).
- Fissure burs: designing a block that is subsequently removed with a bone rongeur or with chisels (Fig 8-4).
- Running 4/0 resorbable sutures can be used for closing (Fig 8-5).

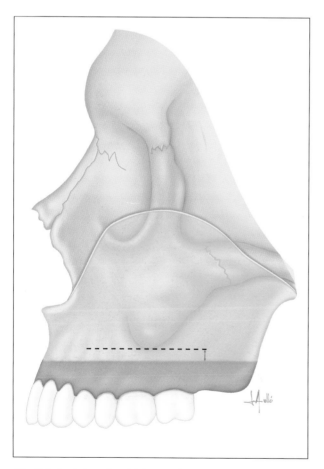

Fig 8-1 Incision should be made over the mucogingival junction.

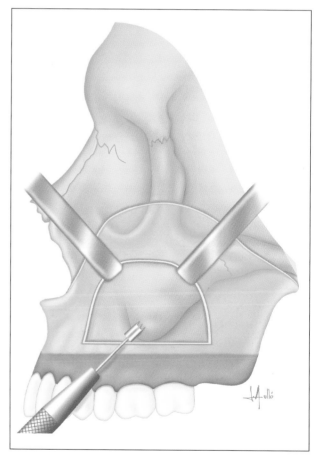

Fig 8-2 Trephining constitutes a very easy and fast harvesting procedure.

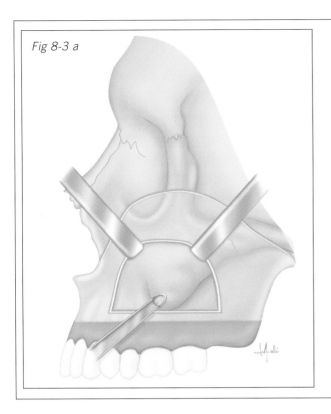

Fig 8-3 a

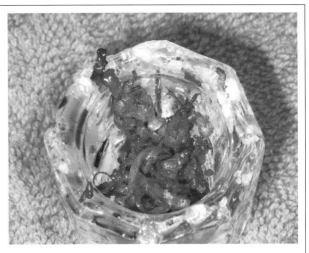

Fig 8-3 b

Fig 8-3 (a, b) The bone scrapper allows harvesting of bone shavings very effectively. This type of graft is suitable for small cavities and three-wall defects.

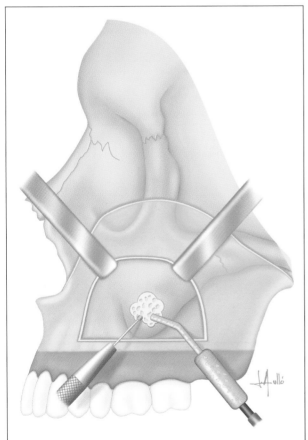

Fig 8-4 Grinding the area with a bur and collecting the particles with a bone filter is also useful.

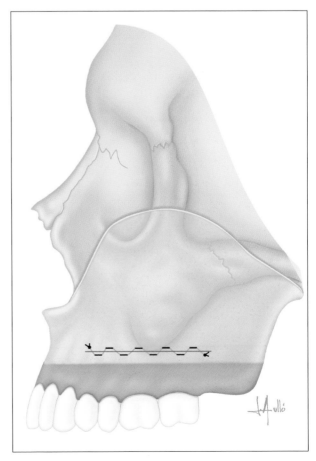

Fig 8-5 Closure with a running suture.

Complications

Neural: Excessive traction or compression of the infraorbital nerve can produce transient or prolonged paraesthesia of the cheek.

Sinusal: Perforation of the sinus membrane will not have effects in the majority of cases. However, in cases with a concomitant sinus lift procedure, membrane preservation is essential.

Trismus: Strippping of the masseter muscle from the ZB may produce transient masticatory dysfunction. When fibres are transected it is advisable to inject corticosteroids locally.

Clinical Applications

ZB harvesting can be used for minor defects, such as the covering of exposed implant threads, vestibular augmentation and alveolar regeneration post-extraction (Fig 8-6a-j).

Fig 8-6 (a-j) Bone grafting from the buttress with a trephine. A sinus lift is done concomitantly and the trephined bone is milled and mixed with bovine inorganic matrix and PRP and used to graft the sinus. Adding some autologous bone to any reconstruction adds osteogenic and osteoinductive potential.

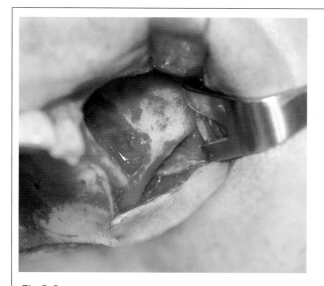

Fig 8-6 a

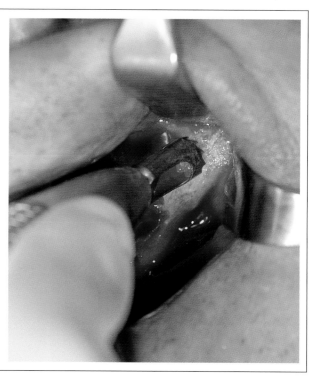

Fig 8-6 b

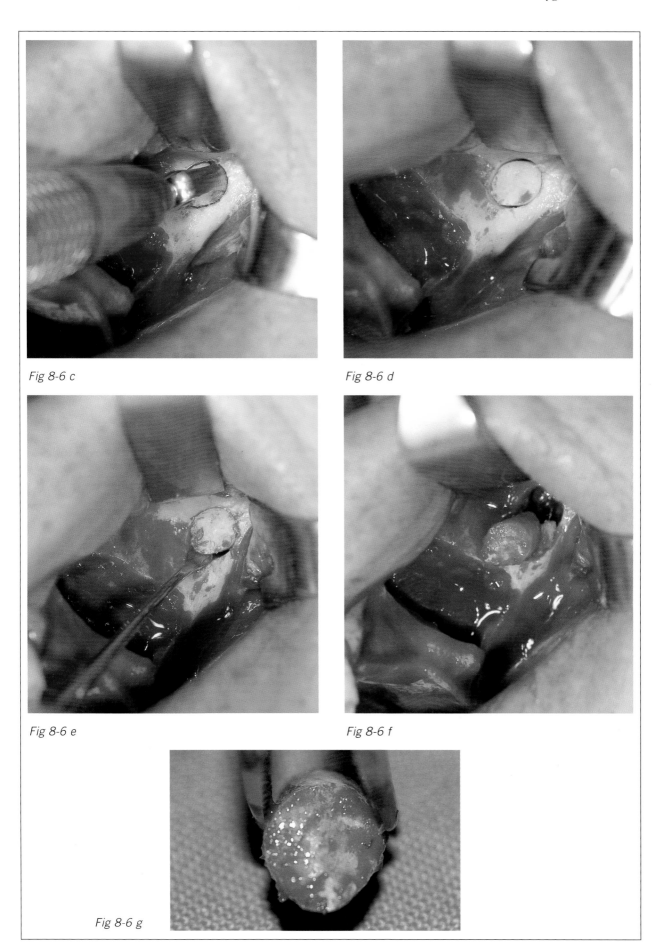

Fig 8-6 c

Fig 8-6 d

Fig 8-6 e

Fig 8-6 f

Fig 8-6 g

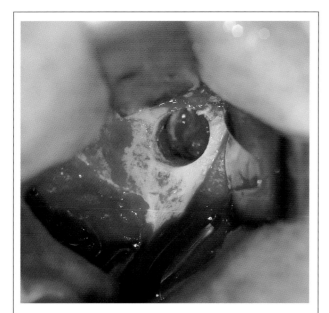

Fig 8-6 h

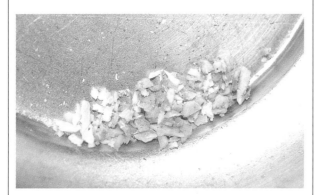

Fig 8-6 i

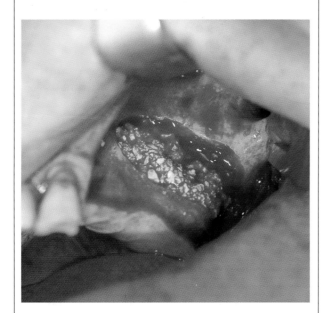

Fig 8-6 j

References

1   Kainulainen VT, Sandor GK, Oikarinen KS, Clokie CM. Zygomatic bone: An additional donor site for alveolar bone reconstruction. Technical note. Int J Oral Maxillofac Implants 2002;17:723-728.

2   Marentette LJ, Maisel RH. Three-dimensional CT reconstruction in midfacial surgery. Otolaryngol Head Neck Surg 1988;98:48-52.

Chapter 9

Calvarium

Surgical Anatomy

The use of the calvarium as a potential bone donor site was initially suggested by Koning and Mullere in 1890. The first recorded surgical approach was performed by Dandy in 1929.[1] Nevertheless, widespread use of calvarial bone grafts in craniomaxillofacial reconstruction was due to the expertise of Paul Tessier.[2,3] Parietal grafts provide material for bony defects, onlays and inlays in several surgical procedures - Le Fort, midface onlay graft and mandibular grafts and continuity defects.

Parietal bone is even and symmetric, situated next to the cranial vertex and together forming the upper calvarium. The ossification is membranous, and growing and remodelling occurs by apposition of new layers through the periosteum at the upper surface and simultaneous osteoclastic resorption from the under-surface. Several authors have demonstrated that bone grafts of membranous bone origin resorb significantly less than endochondral bone grafts (for instance, iliac crest, rib or tibia).[4-9] Other authors related the different embryological origin to a prompt vascularisation (Whitaker, Zins).[10,11] Nevertheless, current hypotheses (Hardesty y Marsh) [12] consider the micro-architecture the cause for difference in resorption. Membranous bones tend to have thick and dense cortical plates and a thin and compact cancellous areas compared to endochondral bones. Ozaki and Buchman[13] demonstrated that cortical bone grafts resorb less than cancellous ones. Chen et al[14] also demonstrated that the cancellous part of the grafts suffer an important neovascularisation, with high osteoclastic activity resulting in high degrees of resorption.

Both parietal bones articulate together in the midline through the sagittal suture, and with the frontal bone through the coronal suture, in the posterior line with the occipital bone through the lambdoid suture and lateral and inferiorly with the temporal bone and the major sphenoidal wing. The outer surface of the bone is covered with part of the temporoparietal fascia, the anteroinferior part of the temporal muscle and above them the scalp. Tightly adhering to the under-surface is the dura. The superior longitudinal sinus underlies the sagittal suture.

The parietal bone consists of the inner and outer cortices with a cancellous layer called diploe (sometimes quite thin) in between.

Surgical Procedure

Calvarial bone grafts are best harvested from the parietal region and seldom from the frontal or occipital areas (Fig 9-1). Whenever possible the bone over the non-dominant hemisphere should be chosen. The temporal area has to be avoided because the calvarium is thinner with no diploe. The mean parietal thickness is 7.45mm ± 1.03mm (from 4mm to 12mm). A CT scan might help in calculating the thickness of the bone and the presence or absence of diploe.[15]

The patient is placed face up, with the head hyperextended and slightly tilted to the opposite side of the donor region. Bone-graft harvesting can be done under local anaesthesia plus sedation, although general anaesthesia is commonly used.

Splits of the outer cortex, full-thickness outer cortex, bicortical or inner cortex grafts are the most common techniques for parietal bone graft harvesting. Osteoperiosteal grafts (thin but easy to reshape) or scrapings of the outer bone surface, which provide useful amounts of bone powder for cavity filling or alveolar edge defects, are also used.

The use of the parietal bone graft as a pedicled flap to the temporoparietal fascia (through the superficial temporal artery and vein) is limited to large maxillofacial defects.[16-18]

The most common donor area within the parietal bone is the temporal tuberosity. However, it is possible to use the occipitoparietal region if we require straight grafts or larger amounts of bone.[15] A safety margin of at least 20mm lateral to the sagittal suture should be maintained because the dura is tightly adherent to the under-surface of the bone, and the underlying sagittal sinus might be damaged in the case of elevation of the inner cortex.

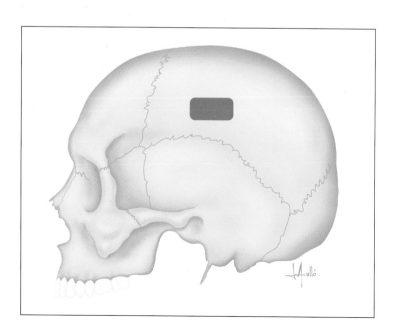

Fig 9-1 Parietal bone from the non-dominant side has the best quality/safety ratio among the various calvarial bones.

Regarding surgical approaches, a longitudinal antero-posterior scalp incision is commonly used, although horizontal or 'T-Y' incisions can also be used. Hair is rarely shaved in preparation for graft harvesting (Fig 9-2 a, b). Previous hair-washing with a chlorhexidine solution instead of iodinate solution is preferred. Five minutes before the scalp incision an infiltration with 2% lidocaine and 1:100 000 epinephrine solution is recommended. Cranial and oral surgical fields are dressed separately, and different instrumentation must be used.

An incision of less than 50mm usually suffices. A No.10 or 23 blade is used to cut the skin, followed by an electric scalpel once the hair follicles are left behind. Whenever possible, cauterisation should be made with bipolar forceps, avoiding scalp clamps and using the autostatic retractor to keep tension at the incision edges, thus collapsing small vessels (Fig 9-3 a, b). The parietal bone surface is exposed with a periosteal elevator. It is important to reflect the periosteal layer in order to minimise postoperative discomfort and oedema (Fig 9-4). The graft is out-

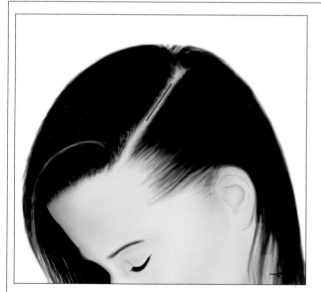

Fig 9-2 a

Fig 9-2 (a, b) It is not necessary to shave the hair at the donor area. Combing the hair bilaterally and designing a 50-70mm line is sufficient to gain access to the area.

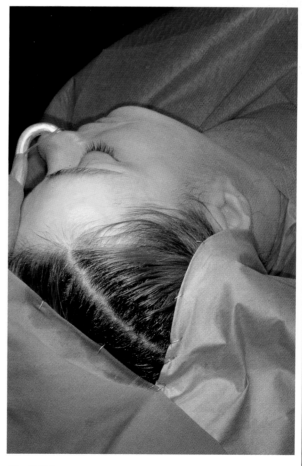

Fig 9-2 b

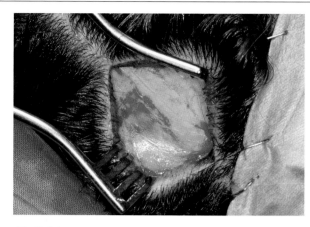

Fig 9-3 b

Fig 9-3 a

Fig 9-3 (a, b) An orthostatic retractor develops a squared surgical field. It maintains the small arteries in the soft tissue in a collapsed form, thus avoiding excessive bleeding during the procedure.

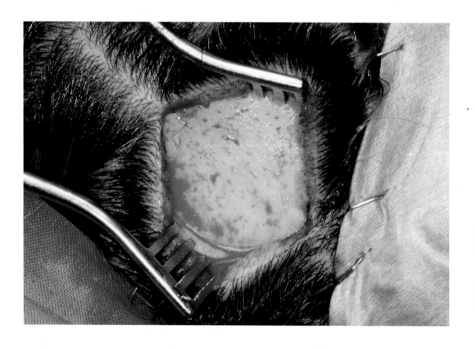

Fig 9-4 It is essential to reflect the periosteum before performing the osteotomies. This layer will protect the donor site after the procedure.

lined with a small sagittal saw or with a fissure bur (Fig 9-5 a, b), the latter causing higher bone waste but permitting easier access for the osteotome parallel to the inner cortex.[19, 20] Osteotomy should stop when the diploic space is reached, indicated by bone bleeding.

The cutting edge of a wide sharp osteotome should proceed parallel to the outer and inner cortices within the diploic space advancing carefully to elevate the graft (Fig 9-6 a-c). Attempts to harvest large grafts (larger than 40mm) often result in fracture during graft removal, as well as increasing the risk of intracraneal exposure (11% of cases). The surgeon should consider the use of multiple small grafts whenever possible.

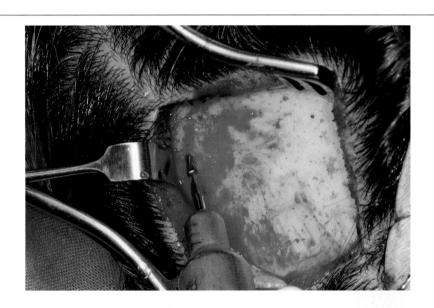

Fig 9-5 a

Fig 9-5 b

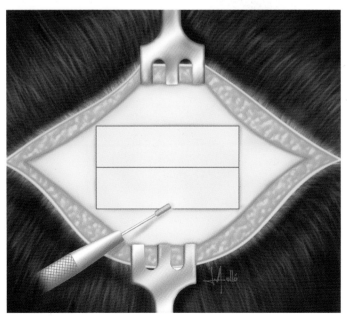

Fig 9-5 (a, b) Fissure burs are very useful in designing the osteotomies since they give sensitive control of the depth. It is important to avoid penetration into the inner cortex to avoid dural tears.

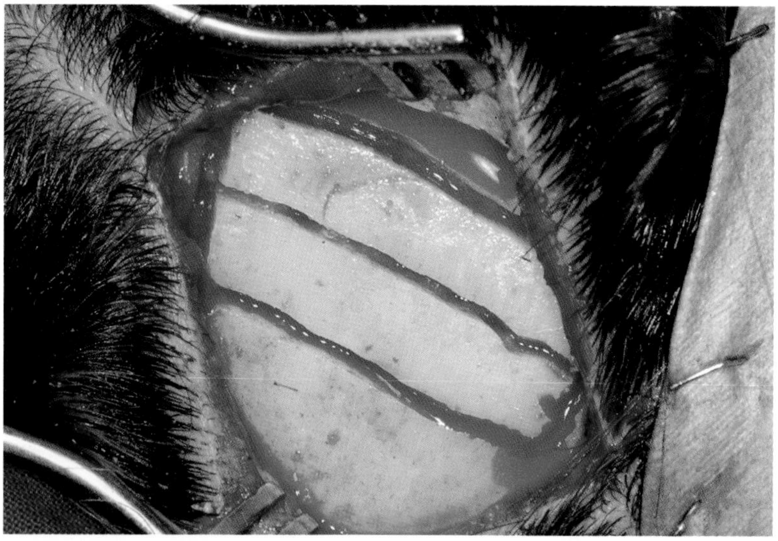

Fig 9-6 a

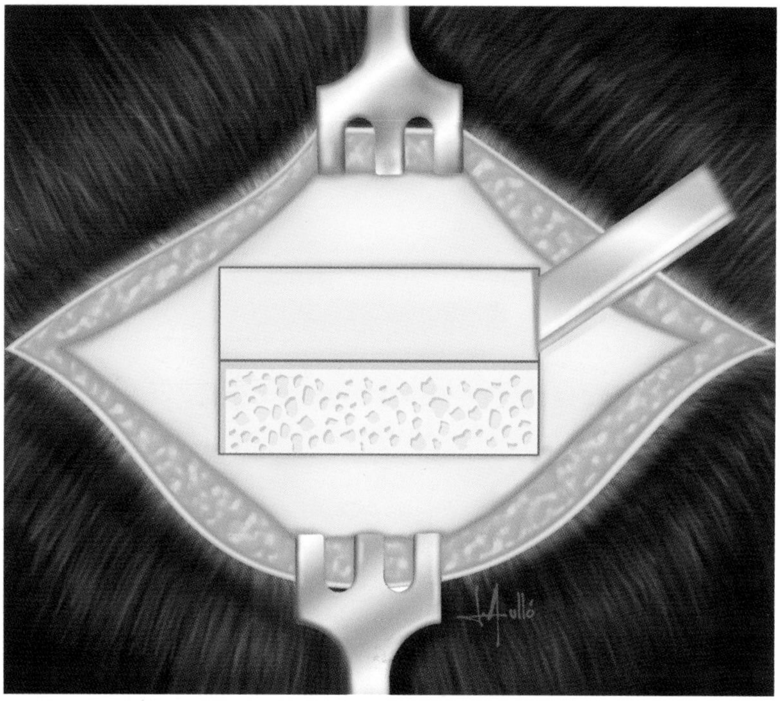

Fig 9-6 b

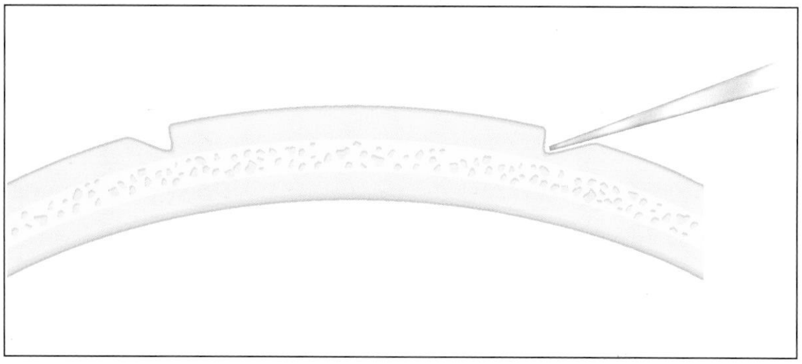

Fig 9-6 c

Fig 9-6 (a-c) Elevation of the blocks is achieved with osteotomes acting parallel to the grafts. This facilitates cutting through the diploic space, thus reducing the risk of graft fracture.

Small amounts of cancellous bone can further be obtained by curettage after removal of the inner cortex (Fig 9-7). If bleeding at the donor site is detected, cauterisation with an electric scalpel and the placing of haemostatic materials, such as Surgicel® instead of bone wax,[21] is recommended (Fig 9-8). The incision is closed with resorbable sutures for the deep periosteal plane, and staples for the skin and subcutaneous tissue (Fig 9-9 a, b). Either a suction drainage or cranial compressive bandage is applied for 24 hours.

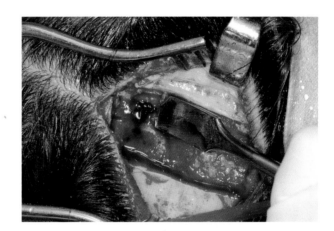

Fig 9-7 Small amounts of cancellous bone can be peeled off the inner cortex once the outer blocks have been removed.

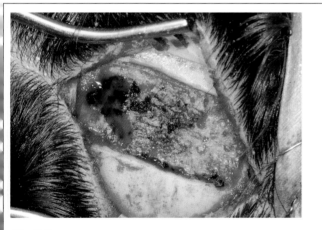

Fig 9-8 a

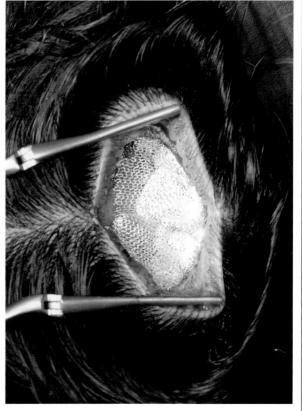

Fig 9-8 (a, b) Haemostasis can be achieved by electric cautery, bone wax or resorbable collagen.

Fig 9-8 b

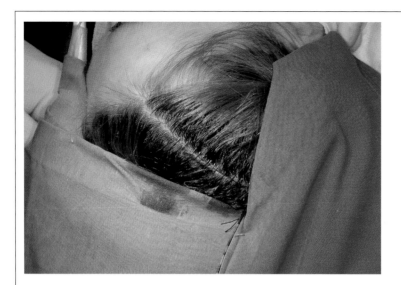

Fig 9-9 a

Fig 9-9 b

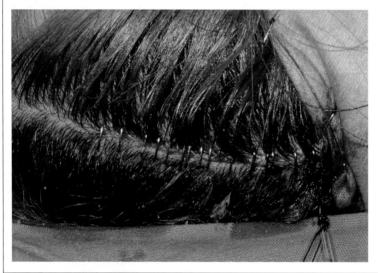

Fig 9-9 (a, b) Closing of the incision is done in two layers. The deep periosteal layer is important to protect the donor area and facilitate bone regeneration. The subcutaneous-superficial layer is best done with staples, since they compress the flaps and are easy to remove.

Parietal bone grafts can also be harvested with a Gigli saw.[22] In these cases, larger bone exposition and pericraneal soft tissue retraction is required. The advantages of this technique are:

- Easier harvesting of larger grafts.
- Shorter surgical time.
- Lower risk of graft fracture.
- Almost complete avoidance of the risk of entering through the inner cortex.

Disadvantages are:

- Larger bone exposition and soft tissue retraction
- Longer training time for acquiring expertise

The bone graft can be associated with the temporoparietal fascia to obtain a pediculated osteofascial flap with the superficial temporal artery and vein pedicle, useful in cases with poor mucosal coverage.[16-18,23]

The parietal and other calvarial bone regions can serve to extract a bone paste by scrapping the bone surface trough a small stab incision and undermining of the periosteal layer. This bony paste either alone or combined with PRP can be used to fill cystic cavities or alveolar layers.

Clinical Applications

Parietal bone blocks can be used for a number of situations as veneer, saddle or interpositional grafts. Cortex scrapings may also be harvested with minimal trauma still yielding enough material for a small sinus lift (Fig 9-10 and 9-11).

Bone parietal advantages are:[24]
- Slow resorption.[14]
- High stability for osteointegration.[25]

- Proximity between donor and recipient sites and common embryological origin.
- Low morbidity at donor site.
- Easy screw fixation.
- Harvesting of large grafts is possible.
- Minimal postsurgical discomfort and short hospitalisation.

Disadvantages are:
- Thinner grafts.
- Visible scars in patients with alopecia.
- Difficult modelling with risk of fracture.
- Higher risk of dura injury during exposure.
- Longer surgical time.

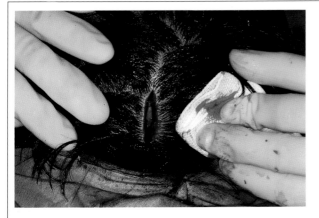

Fig 9-10 a

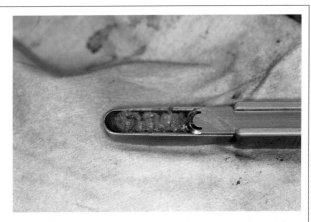

Fig 9-10 b

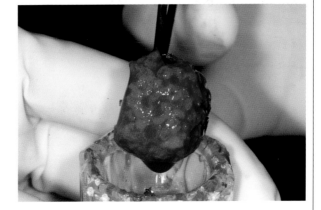

Fig 9-10 c

Fig 9-10 (a-c) A stab incision allows limited periosteal elevation and harvesting of bone shavings with the aid of a bone scrapper. Small to mid-sized three-wall defects can be reconstructed with particulated bone from this site.

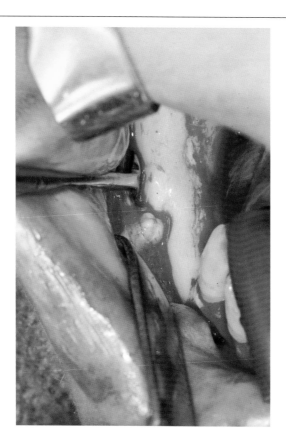

Fig 9-11 (a) A young woman presenting with bilateral posterior mandibular atrophy. Iliac crest was initially proposed as donor site. The patient refused this approach because of 'visible' scars. Parietal bone was suggested as the alternative. The vertical defect at the right side is depicted in the image. Note how the nerve has been identified.

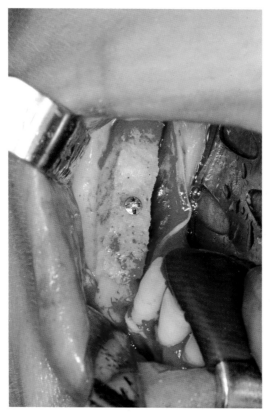

Fig 9-11 (b) Reconstruction with a long block from the parietal region.

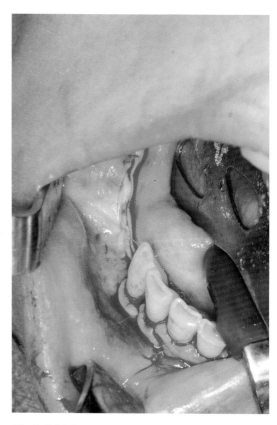

Fig 9-11 (c) Watertight and tension-free closure is a must to avoid exposure of the graft.

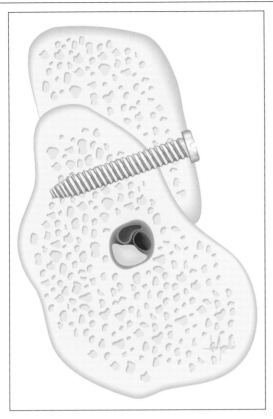

Fig 9-11 d

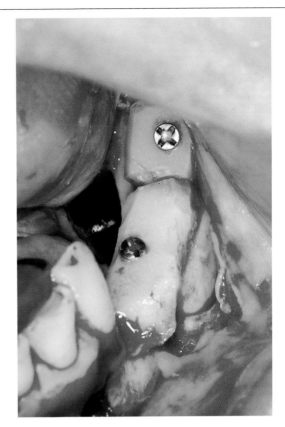

Fig 9-11 e

Fig 9-11 (d, e) The contralateral side was reconstructed with two saddle grafts from the same area, each of them fixed with a screw.

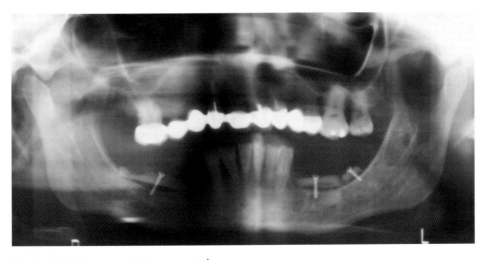

Fig 9-11 (f) Panoramic X-ray control.

It is difficult to convince patients to allow harvesting from the head when it comes to oral pre-prosthetic reconstruction.

Complications

Parietal bone graft harvesting has a low rate of complications. In a study of over 12,672 parietal bone grafts, performed by Kline and Wolfe,[26] the reported rate of complications was 0.18% (23 cases). Dura exposure was not reported among the complications, although it occurred in 11% of the cases. Reported complications were surgical wound infections, dural injuries and exceptionally transitory neurological defects.

In comparison, complications in iliac crest bone grafts vary from 3% *(Kline and Wolfe)* to 20% of the cases *(Marx, Morales, Laurie et al)*. In our experience, morbidity from calvarium harvesting compares favourably with that of the iliac crest. When outer cortex bony 'chips' harvesting is undertaken through the use of a scrapper, complications are extremely rare. Prompt identification and treatment of eventual complications is crucial. In cases of dura exposure, the region should be covered with a graft. Dural lacerations are dealt with by first extending the craniotomy beyond the limits of the tear. If injury is found, neurosurgical consultation is indicated.

In relation to cranial bone defects, patients are tolerant of donor-site depression as long as the bone edges are not too sharp (sometimes filling the donor area with bony chips is recommended).

References

1   Dandy WE. An operative treatment for certain cases of meningoceles (or encephalocele) into the orbit. Arch Ophthalmol1929;2:123.

2   Tessier P. Autogenous bone grafts taken from the calvarium for facial and cranial applications. Clin Plast Surg 1982;9:531-538.

3   Tessier P. Aesthetic aspects of bone grafting to the face. Clin Plast Surg 1981;8:279-302.

4   Jackson IT, Pellett C, Smith JM. The skull as a bone graft donor site. Ann Plast Surg 1983;11:527-532.

5   Hemar P, Herman D, Piller P, et al. Results of the use of parietal bone as bone graft donor site in facial reconstruction: Apropos of 71 cases. Ann Chir Plast Esthet 1995;40:349-356.

6   Siddique S, Mathog R. A comparison of parietal and iliac crest bone grafts for orbital reconstruction. J Oral Maxillofac Surg 2002;60:44-50.

7   Hunter D, Baker S, Sobol SM. Split calvarial grafts in maxillofacial reconstruction. Otolaryngol Head Neck Surg 1990;102:345-350.

8   Donovan MG, Dickerson NC, Hellstein JW, Hanson LJ. Autologous calvarial and iliac onlay bone grafts in miniature swine. J Oral Maxillofac Surg 1993;51:898-903.

9   Harsa BC, Turvey TA, Powers SK. Use of autogenous cranial bone grafts in maxillofacial surgery: A preliminary report. J Oral Maxillofac Surg 1986;44:11-15.

10 Zins J, Whitaker LA. Membranous versus encondral bone: Implications for craneofacial reconstruction. Plast Rec Surg 1983;72:778-785.

11 Zins JE, Kusiak JF, Whitaker LA, et al. The influence of the recipient site on bone grafts to the face. Plast Rec Surg 1984;73:371-381.

12 Hardesty RA, Marsh GL. Craneofacial onlay bone grafting: A prospective evaluation of graft morfology, orientation and embryologic origin. Plast Rec Surg 1990; 85:5-14.

13 Ozaki W, Buchman SR, Goldstein SA, Fyhrie DP. A comparative analysis of the microarchitecture of cortical membranous and cortical endochondral onlay bone grafts in the craneofacial esqueleton. Plast Rec Surg 1999;104:139-147.

14 Chen NJ, Glowacki JG, Bucky LP, et al. The roles of revascularization and resorption on endurance of craniofacial onlay bone grafts in the rabbit. Plast Rec Surg 1994;93:714-719.

15 Pensler J, Mc Carthy J. The calvarial donor site: An anatomic study in cadavers. Plast Rec Surg 1985;75:648-651.

16 Musolas A, Colombini E, Michelena J. Vascularized full-thickness bone grafts in Maxillofacial reconstruction: The role of the galea and superficial temporal vessels. Plast Rec Surg 1991;87:261-267.

17 Undt G, Hollmann K, Schuster H, Rasse M. Pedicled calvarial bone flap for reconstruction of the anterior skull base following tumour resection. Plast Rec Surg 1996;98:730-734.

18 Piller P, Herman D, Kennel P, et al. Transfert osseux vascularise en ìlot de los parietal. Ann Chir Plat Esthet 1993;38:532-541.

19 Bell WH. Modern Practice in Orthognathic and Reconstructive Surgery. Philadelphia, PA: WB Saunders Co, 1992.

20 Frodel JL, Marentette LJ, Quatela VC, et al. Cranial bone graft harvest, techniques, considerations and morbidity. Arch Otolaryngol Head Neck Surg 1993;119:17.

21 Thaller SR, Kim S, Tesluk H, Kawamoto H. The split calvarial bone graft donor site: The effects of surgical and hidroxyapatite impregnated with collagen. Ann Plast Surg 1990;26:435-439.

22 Stevens M, Heit J. Calvarial bone grafting using the Gigli saw. J Oral Maxillofac Surg 1998;56:798-799.

23 Gratz KW, Salier HF, Haers PE, Oeschslin Ck, Mandibular reconstruction with full thickness calvarial bone and temporal muscle flap. Br J Oral Maxillofac Surg 1996;34:379-385.

24 Tessier P. Complications associated with the harvesting of cranofacial bone graft (discussion). Plast Rec Surg 1995;95:14-20.

25 Orsini G, Bianchi A, Vinci R, Piattelli A. Histologic evaluation of autogenous calvarial bone in maxillary onlay bone grafts: A report of 2 cases. Int J Oral Maxillofac Implants 2003;18 594-598.

26 Kline RM, Wolfe AS. Complications associated with the harvesting of cranial bone grafts. Plast Rec Surg 1995;95:5-13.

27 Marx RE, Morales MJ. Morbidity from bone harvest in major jaw construction. J Oral Maxillofac Surg 1988;46:196.

163

Iliac Crest

Surgical Anatomy

The iliac crest (IC) has been widely used for major reconstructions in the maxillofacial area.[1,2] Its use in preprosthetic surgery has been advocated for different clinical situations (Fig 10-1 a-d).[3-8] Nowadays, we save this site for instances where large amounts of cortico-cancellous bone are required (Fig10-2 a, b).[9] When only cancellous bone is required we favour the use of the tibia as a donor site [10], and if small blocks are needed (for instance, for up to four missing teeth) we can obtain them from intraoral sources as previously described.

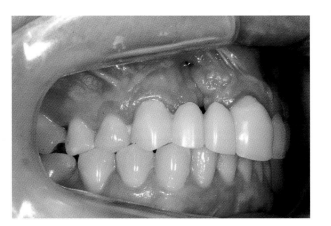

Fig 10-1 (a) Congenital cleft.

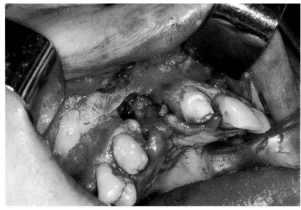

Fig 10-1 (b) Surgical approach showing bone defect, after reconstruction of the nasal floor.

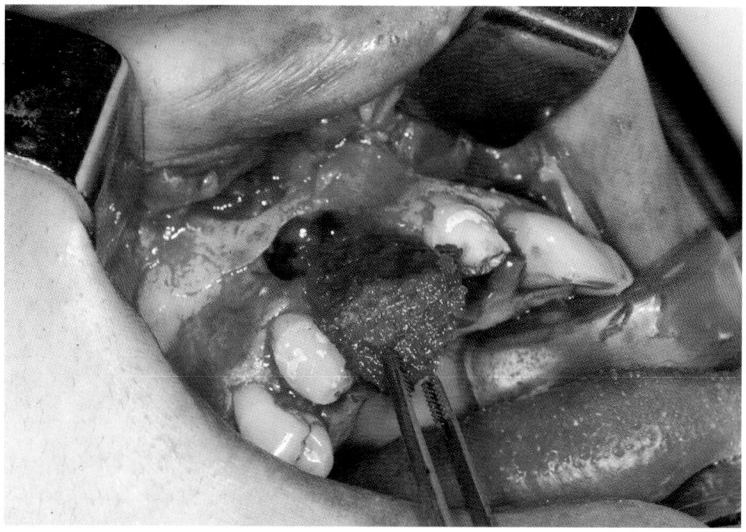

Fig 10-1 c

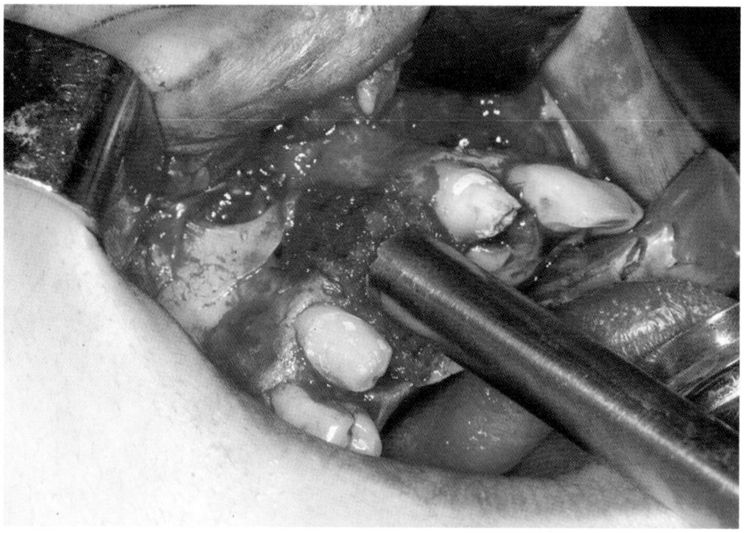

Fig 10-1 d

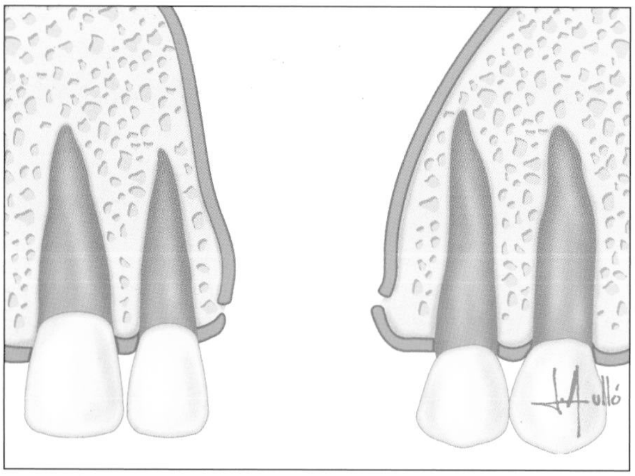

Fig 10-1 e

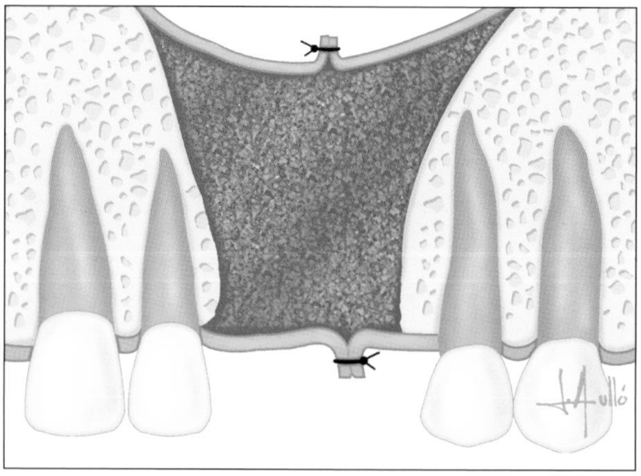

Fig 10-1 f

Fig 10-1 (c-f) Block of cancellous bone harvested from the anterior iliac crest is impacted in the defect. For years the iliac crest has been the donor site of choice even for moderate defects.

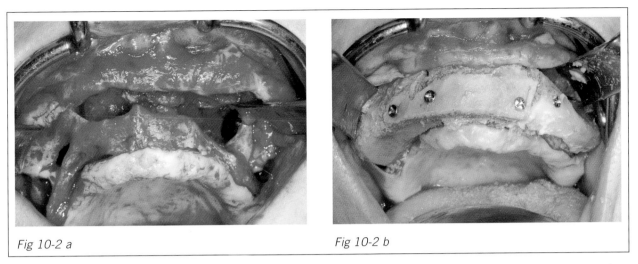

Fig 10-2 a

Fig 10-2 b

Fig 10-2 (a, b) Severe maxillary atrophy reconstructed with several corticocancellous blocks in an attempt to restore a normal anatomical situation.

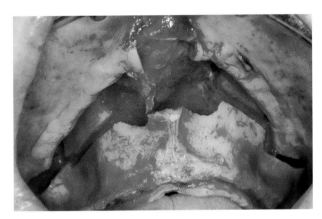

Fig 10-2 (c) Total maxillary atrophy with class IV anteriorly and class VI posteriorly. Reconstruction is done via Le Fort I osteotomy for downgrafting.

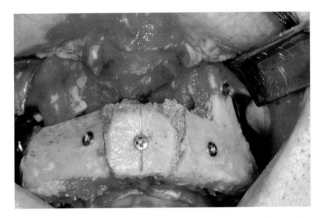

Fig 10-2 (d) Inlay grafts on the sinus floor bilaterally and blocks at the anterior maxilla in a veneer fashion. Note how the block on the left side acts as a stabilising plate, maintaining the new vertical position of the reconstructed maxilla.

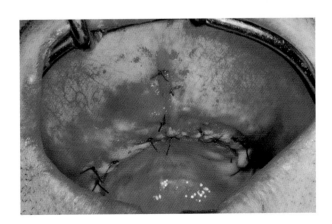

Fig 10-2 (e) Watertight suture of the flaps is mandatory to preserve a sealed situation for the reconstruction.

However, there are a number of instances were severe maxillo-mandibular atrophy leaves the IC as the only possible source of grafts (Fig 10-3 a-c).

Bone grafts from the iliac crest are endochondral in origin. The ala of the ilium is smoothly concave on the pelvic surface and convex on the gluteal surface. The anterosuperior and postero-superior iliac spine constitute the limits of the crest.

Approximately 50mm behind the anterosuperior spine is a prominent tubercle. Because the anterior ilium is thickest between the antero-superior spine and the tubercle, these are important landmarks.[11]

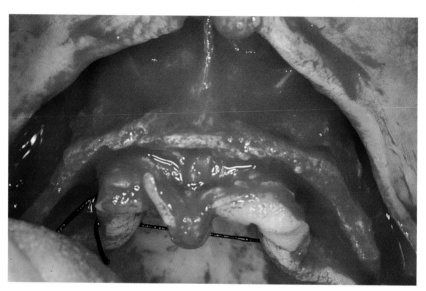

Fig 10-3 (a) Class IV atrophy with adequate height yet insufficient width of the crest. In such a case, the only choices for bone harvesting are iliac crest or calvarial.

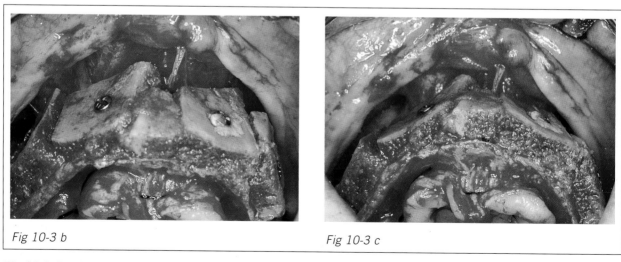

Fig 10-3 b   *Fig 10-3 c*

Fig 10-3 (b, c) Corticocancellous blocks from IC allow adequate reconstruction of the atrophied maxilla.

Both anatomically and surgically the IC can be divided into anterior and posterior. Although the posterior IC yields higher amounts of bone,[12] surgical access to this site necessitates a positional change in the patient, making it impossible to work simultaneously at the donor and recipient area and thus increasing surgical time.

The anterior IC is the donor site of choice in most cases because during maxillofacial reconstructions patients are usually in a supine position.

In most instances the anterior IC suffices for preprosthetic maxillofacial reconstruction.

Available bone at the IC is located behind the anterior spine. Caudally, the iliac crest gets thinner and the two cortical layers approach each other, leaving a scarce amount of cancellous bone between them. This anatomical situation explains why grafts from this site have an inverted pyramid shape with the base at the upper part (Fig 10-4). The mean size of blocks harvested from this site varies between 50-60mm in length and 30-40mm in width. The thickness varies from the upper part at 20-30mm to the lower part at 0-10mm. In terms of volume between 30cc and 50cc of corticocancellous bone can be obtained.[12]

When harvesting bone from any site, one of the goals is obtaining the maximum amount of bone with the lowest morbidity. This is particularly true in this area where postoperative discomfort constitutes the main drawback.

Morbidity at this area depends on amount of blood loss, sensory disturbances and transient or permanent muscular injury.

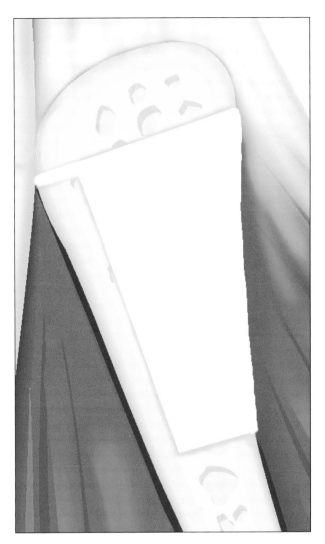

Fig 10-4 The shape of the iliac crest allows harvesting of pyramidal bone blocks.

To reduce this side-effect as much as possible a thorough understanding of regional anatomy is essential, and a careful technique should be followed.

There are some important anatomical relationships (Fig 10-5):

The lateral cutaneous branch of the iliohipogastric nerve - this crosses the crest posterior and superior to the anterior spine and innervates the lateral anterior portion of the iliac crest.

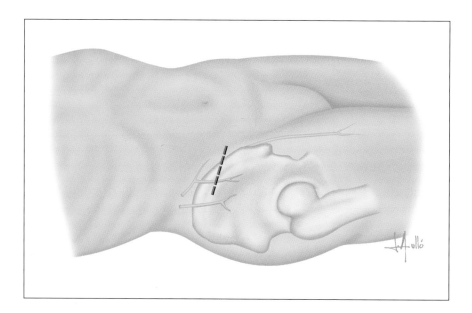

Fig 10-5 Understanding the path of the nerves in the area is of utmost importance to minimise morbidity.

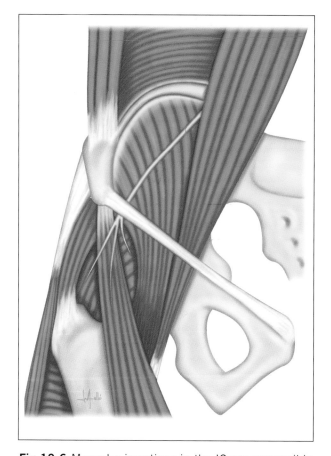

Fig 10-6 Muscular insertions in the IC are responsible for most of the postoperative disturbances.

The lateral branch of the subcostal nerve - this crosses the crest over the anterior spine and innervates the lateral–inferior portion of the crest.

The lateral femoral cutaneous nerve - this crosses the anterosuperior spine under the inguinal ligament, although occasionally it may cross over the spine. This nerve is by far the most frequently affected by IC harvesting procedures.

Morbidity in removal of IC grafts is due primarily to damage to either the gluteus medius or the gluteus maximus muscle. Because of this, patients experience discomfort and gait disturbances for a variable period after surgery.

The iliac muscle inserts medially at the anterior portion of the crest. Internal, external oblique and transverse muscles insert medially on the crest. Finally the minor, medius and maximus gluteal muscles are inserted at the lateral aspect of the crest (Fig 10-6).

Surgical Procedure

Position

The patient is placed in the supine position. A rolled towel is placed beneath the buttock to elevate and slightly rotate the anterior iliac crest. The surgical field is decontaminated with iodine and a sterile drape is applied (Fig 10-7).

Anaesthesia

Hypotensive general anaesthesia is usually recommended for iliac crest harvesting, unless a minimally invasive approach is planned to obtain only cancellous bone or bone marrow. Nasotracheal intubation is advisable to ease access to the oral cavity for the reconstructive phase of the surgery.

Access

Following isolation of the field the anterosuperior iliac spine, crest and tubercle are palpated. By firmly pressing medial and superior to these landmarks, the skin may be pulled over the crest (Fig 10-8). Doing so, the incision will fall away from the bony prominences and belt line and within the area of the swimsuit. Medial incisions[13] and incisions on natural abdominal creases can be made in selected cases. The incision should start 20mm posterior to the spine and should be parallel to the anterosuperior part of the crest. The length must not exceed 50mm (Fig 10-9), thereby avoiding severing the femorocutaneous nerve.

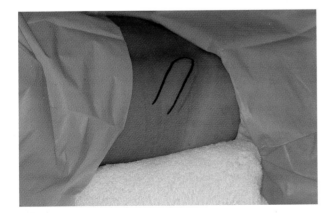

Fig 10-7 With the patient in supine position, a rolled towel is positioned under the buttock and the bony landmarks identified.

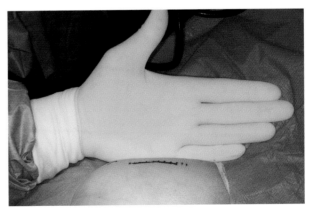

Fig 10-8 Pressing the skin medially, the incision is placed over the crest. This trick will prevent severing of the nerve and will place the future scar away from the belt line.

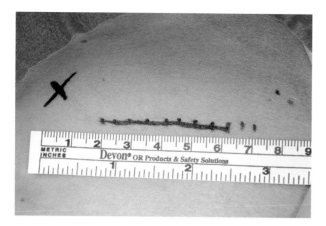

Fig 10-9 In this image, the X marks the anterosuperior spine. Incision should start at least 20mm behind the spine, and the length should not exceed 50mm.

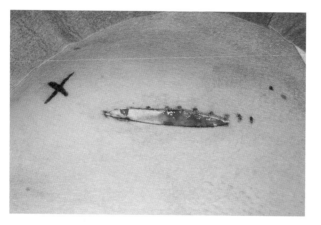

Fig 10-10 A through-and-through incision is done either with a No. 23 blade or with a Colorado needle.

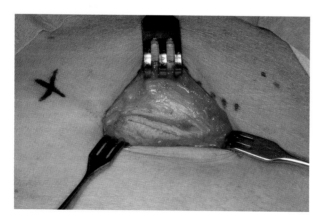

Fig 10-11 The periosteum is then incised longitudinally along the crest.

The incision can be made with either a No. 22 scalpel or with a Colorado needle® (Fig 10-10). The initial incision is carried deeply through subcutaneous tissue to the superficial fascia with an electrical knife. Careful haemostasis should be achieved to avoid chronic oozing from the subcutaneous tissue during the procedure. A white line of periosteum between the gluteal and abdominal muscles is identified, and the incision is continued down to the bone through this area (Fig 10-11). This incision should be 20mm posterior to the anterior iliac spine to avoid damaging the inguinal ligament

Subperiosteal dissection is carried out medially to disinsert oblique and transverse muscles (Fig 10-12 a, b). A wide orthopaedic periosteal elevator will be useful at this stage. Stripping of periosteum at this point may be difficult because of these muscular attachments. The iliacus muscle is stripped from the medial wall to a depth of 100mm. Orthopaedic (Hoffman or Taylor) retractors are inserted at this point to expose the donor site and protect the periosteum and the abdominal cavity (Fig 10-13).

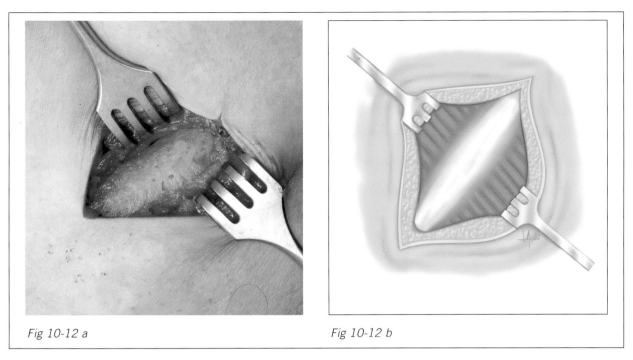

Fig 10-12 a   *Fig 10-12 b*

Fig 10-12 (a, b) De-globing of the crest is done with a wide periosteal elevator. Staying under the periosteum mini-mises muscle disruption, thus lessening postoperative discomfort.

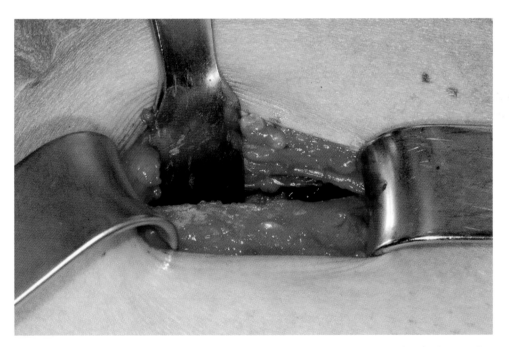

Fig 10-13 Hoffman retractors are very useful in separating the abdominal muscles medially.

Harvesting procedure

• Invasive technique

When corticocancellous blocks are to be obtained there are basically two approaches to gain access to the IC: the 'trap door technique' and the 'split technique'.

– The **'trap door technique'**: In this technique two vertical cuts are made with an oscillating saw 10-20mm through the cortex (Fig 10-14 a-b). These two cuts are connected along the medial surface with the same saw. The crest is then fractured laterally, creating a mobile roof, which hinges at the lateral periosteum and gluteal musculature (Fig 10-15 a-b).

At this point we can obtain harvest cancellous bone or corticocancellous bone, depending on the reconstructive needs.

Cancellous grafts

These can be easily removed with medium-sized orthopaedic curettes, taking care to preserve both medial and lateral cortex. Out-fracturing of the medial cortex with the curettes often occurs and has no relevance. Usually 80-100mm under the crest we will find the limit for our graft harvesting. Below this level the inner and outer cortical layers become closer, and the cancellous bone is scarce. Harvesting can proceed posteriorly under the crest until the amount of desired bone for grafting is collected.

Strictly speaking, if only limited amounts of cancellous bone are to be obtained, this complex approach should not be required. A minimally invasive trephine approach will suffice.

174

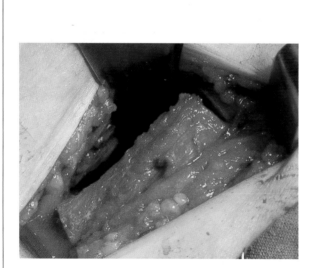

Fig 10-14 a

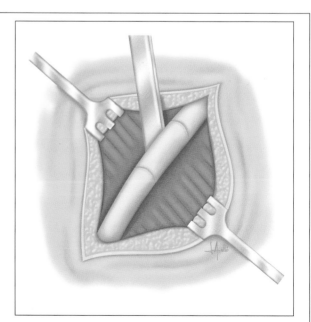

Fig 10-14 b

Fig 10-14 (a, b) In the trap-door technique two vertical osteotomies and one horizontal are connected.

Cortico-cancellous blocks

To obtain a corticocancellous block from the medial side of the ilium, two parallel vertical cuts can be made either with a chisel or with a saw (oscillating or reciprocating) (Fig 10-16 a-b).

Care should be taken to maintain the anterior cut away from the anterior limit of the ilium in order to prevent fracture of the anterior spine. This would result in severe postoperative discomfort for the patient.

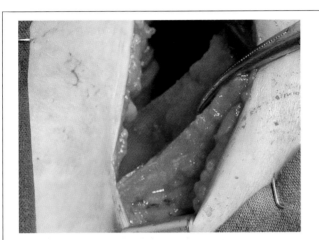

Fig 10-15 a

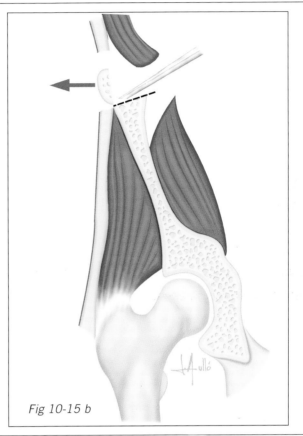

Fig 10-15 b

Fig 10-15 (a, b) The trap door is then pedicled on the lateral periosteal layer and separated laterally.

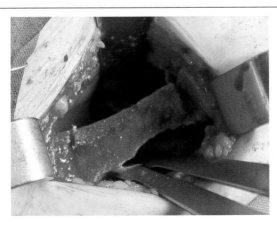

Fig 10-16 a

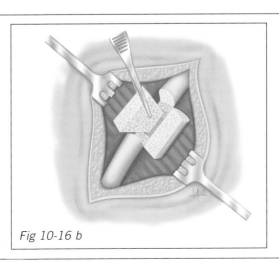

Fig 10-16 b

Fig 10-16 (a, b) One step on each side will provide stable support when the trap door is repositioned.

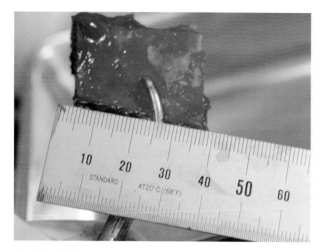

Fig 10-17 Cortico-cancellous block.

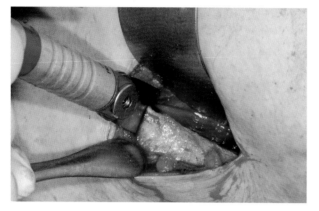

Fig 10-18 In the split technique, lateral continuity of the crest is preserved and the blocks are harvested by osteotomising the medial side of the crest. The vertical cuts are initiated with an oscillating saw.

The inferior portion of these vertical cuts is connected with a horizontal one parallel to the crest. This last cut can be made with an oscillating saw or a curved osteotome. Finally, a wide straight chisel is used to 'peel of' the block from the lateral cortex (Fig 10-17).

– The **'split technique'**: In this technique, again two vertical cuts are made in the crest but leaving intact the lateral half and going downward to a depth equivalent to the width of the desired block (Fig 10-18). Then a longitudinal cut is made, connecting both vertical cuts and going downward to reach the same level as the previous cuts. This is initiated with an oscillating saw and continued with a wide straight chisel (Fig 10-19 a, b).

The inferior portion of these vertical cuts is connected with a horizontal one parallel to the crest. This last cut can be made with an oscillating saw or a curved osteotome.

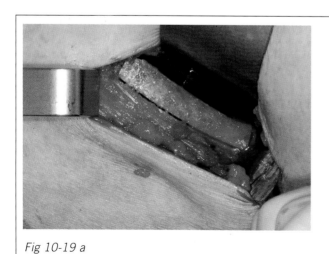

Fig 10-19 a

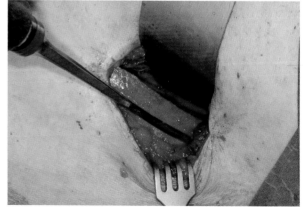

Fig 10-19 b

Fig 10-19 (a, b) Once designed, the osteotomy is completed with wide chisels.

This approach is faster and allows incorporation of the medial section of the crest into the graft. This rounded shape of the graft is extremely useful when vertical reconstruction of the crest is needed (Fig 10-20). Another advantage is that continuity of the crest is not violated (Fig 10-21).

The trap door technique is more time consuming, since the 'roof' has to be repositioned with non-resorbable sutures or wires once the harvesting procedure has been completed (Fig. 10-22). Peeling of the lateral cortex is easier with the trap-door technique, and thus thicker blocks may be obtained.

With both techniques extra cancellous bone can be harvested once the blocks have been removed (Fig 10-23).

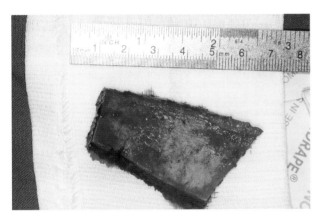

Fig 10-20 Cortico-cancellous block obtained with this technique. The split technique is less traumatic but yields narrower blocks.

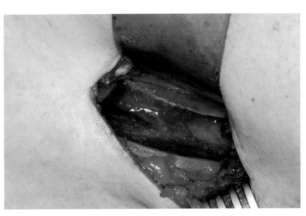

Fig 10-21 Clinical aspect after removal of the block. Note how lateral continuity of the crest is preserved.

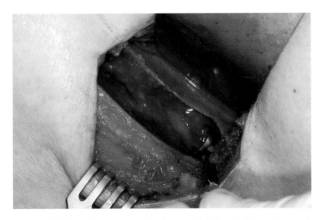

Fig 10-22 A bone curette is useful to further harvest large amounts of cancellous bone once the block has been removed and before closing.

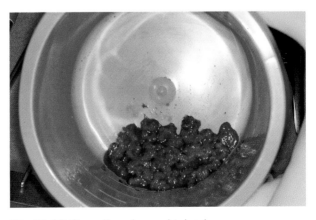

Fig 10-23 Cancellous bone obtained.

Full-thickness grafts from the anterior ilium are rarely needed in preprosthetic surgery. In this case gluteal muscles have to be stripped from the lateral cortex. This will cause more difficulties in ambulation.

• Minimally invasive bone harvest with trephines

Cancellous bone can be removed from the anterior and posterior iliac crest with trephines,[14,15] applying the same principles and technique discussed at the tibia chapter.

Local anaesthesia plus sedation is given in an ambulatory setting.

A 10-20mm stab incision is made down to the iliac crest. A limited periosteal stripping allows application of the trephine against the crest and further perforation of the cortex. Then trephines or curettes can be used for removal of cancellous bone with the aid of a bone filter connected to suction (Fig 10-37).

Closure

Once the desired amount of graft has been obtained, careful haemostasis should follow. Bleeding at the donor site can be stopped with bone wax or a collagenous membrane.[16] The use of external drains is controversial.[17] In our experience they reduce the number of postoperative haematomas and should be left below the periosteal closure (Fig 10-24).

Some authors advocate the use of subperiosteal catheters postoperatively for pain control through injection of local anaesthetic.[18,19]

The trap door should be repositioned and secured in place. We have found that resuturing of periosteum and abdominal muscles to the crest warrants stability of the trap door (Fig 10-25). A trick to facilitate repositioning and stabilisation of the trap door consists of leaving a 'shoulder' of full thickness bone at both sides, on top of which the repositioned segment will rest.

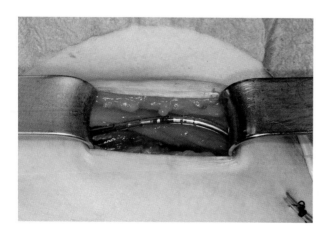

Fig 10-24 A suction drain is placed subperiosteally to reduce the risk of haematoma formation.

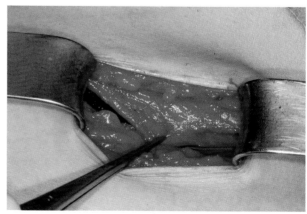

Fig 10-25 Periosteal suture.

The abdominal muscles are sutured to the periosteum on the crest with 2/0 resorbable sutures (Fig 10-26). Then superficial fascia and fat are sutured with the same material (Fig 10-27), the subcutaneous tissues with 3/0 (Fig 10-28), and finally skin with 4/0 intradermal nylon in a running fashion (Fig 10-29).

This last suture will be removed after the 10th day postoperatively.

Postoperative care

A surface compressive dressing is applied and maintained for 48 hours.

No specific limitations for walking are given, although the patient is asked to minimise ambulation for the first 48 hours. The suction drain is removed when it is no longer productive, and hospital discharge usually takes place the day after the procedure.

Some patients require the use of a walking stick for a few days.

Postoperative antibiotics and NSAIDs are prescribed for one week.

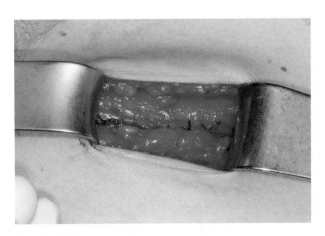

Fig 10-26 Suture of the abdominal muscles.

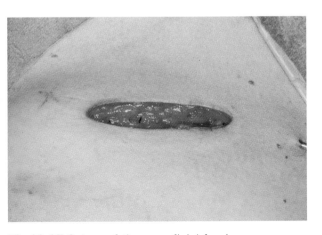

Fig 10-27 Suture of the superficial fascia.

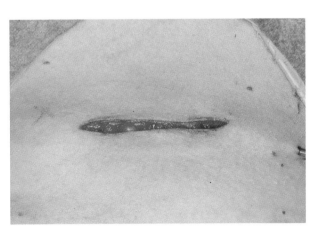

Fig 10-28 Subcutaneous suture.

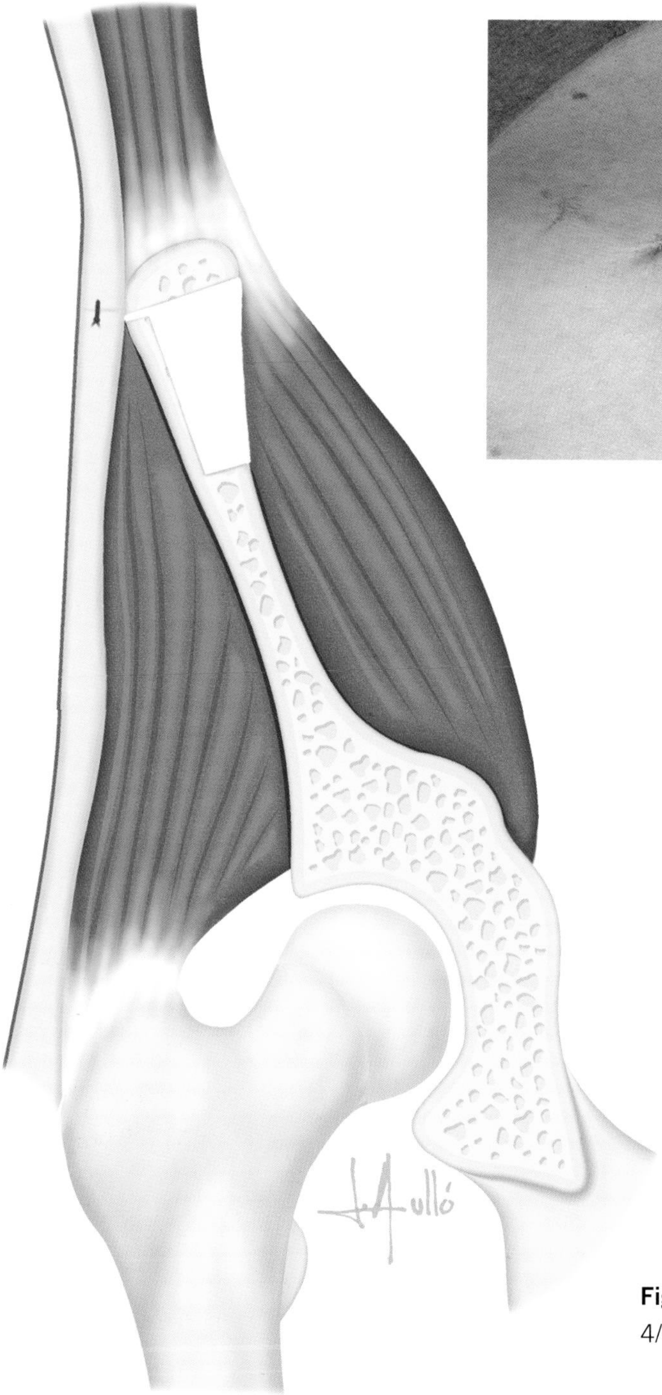

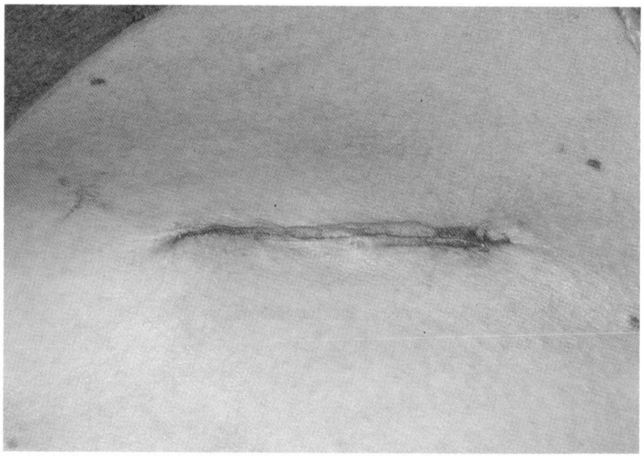

Fig 10-29 Intradermal running suture with 4/0 resorbable monofilament.

Clinical Applications

IC has been the donor site of choice for many years for a number of reconstructive techniques in the maxillofacial region. Its enchondral embryologic origin makes this bone more prone to resorption when compared with bone of membranous origin, but the amount of available material and the high density of bone marrow with stem-cells make this donor site very attractive for major preprosthetic reconstructions.

The IC has been used in virtually all types of maxillomandibular defects.[20-23] However, today we reserve this site for situations where moderate to large blocks are needed. These are severe maxillary atrophy (Fig 10-30, 10-33, 10-34, 10-35), severe mandibular atrophy (Fig 10-35, 10-36) and a combination of partial defects in maxilla and mandible (Fig 10-31, 10-32).

In these situations bone blocks are used as inlay or onlay grafts. Cancellous bone is adequate for sinus lifts using platelet-rich plasma as a carrier.

Complications

Several complications have been described in the literature. However, current technique allows harvesting with low morbidity.[24,25]

Intraoperative

One of the most frequent complications is damage to the cutaneous nerve supply (femorocutaneous) that runs medial to the anterosuperior iliac spine. Care should be taken to place the cutaneous incision below the crest.[26]

Fracture of the anterior spine results in disinsertion of the sartorius muscle. This can also occur during the postoperative period.[27]

Perforation into the abdominal cavity is a rare occurrence.

Postoperative

Most patients will have a noticeable limp, especially in those cases were gluteal muscles have been stripped from the lateral side of the ilium. The duration of the limp will depend on age, gender, physical condition and degree of surgical trauma.[28]

Patients may develop a haematoma, either subcutaneous or retroperitoneal, which should be managed conservatively.[29]

There may be herniation of abdominal contents due to suture dehiscence at the muscular and periosteal level.[30]

Infection is extremely infrequent, since antibiotic prophylaxis is initiated in all patients before surgery.

Unaesthetic scars can be prevented by avoiding cutaneous incisions over the crest and by careful suturing by layers.

181

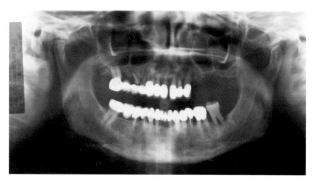

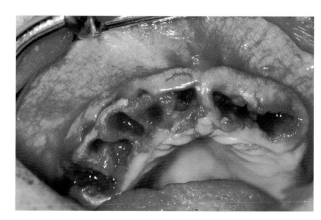

Fig 10-30 (a) Severe periodontal disease in a 50-year-old female with moderate atrophy of the maxilla. Simultaneous removal of remaining teeth and bone reconstruction is planned.

Fig 10-30 (b) Intraoperative view after removal of teeth and curettage of alveoli.

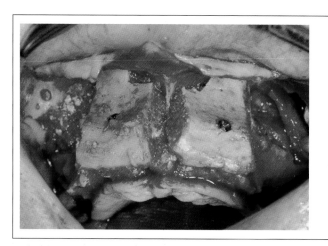

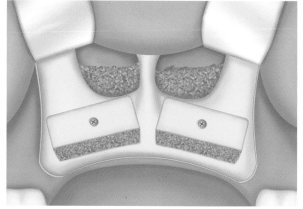

Fig 10-30 (c) Reconstruction of the anterior maxilla with veneer corticocancellous blocks.

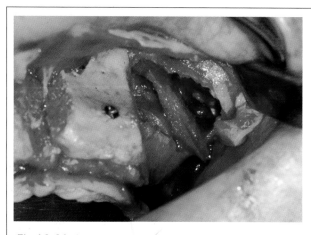

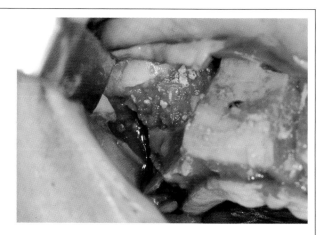

Fig 10-30 d

Fig 10-30 e

Fig 10-30 (d, e) Simultaneous bilateral sinus lift with a roof of cortical bone on each side protecting the sinus membrane and allowing under-compaction of cancellous bone.

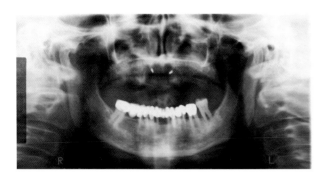

Fig 10-30 (f) Postoperative panoramic X-ray depicting the reconstructed areas.

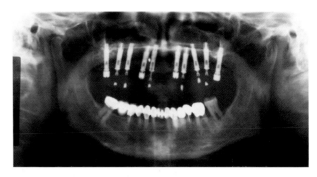

Fig 10-30 (g) Three months after the main procedure, 10 fixtures were placed and six of them immediately loaded.

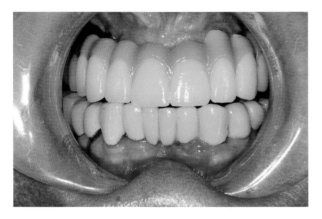

Fig 10-30 (h) Final restoration.

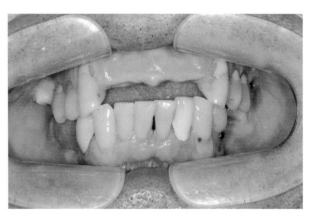

Fig 10-31 (a) Partially edentulous case in the upper and lower with severe periodontal compromise of the molars.

183

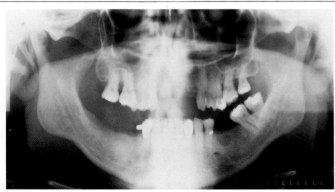

Fig 10-31 b

Fig 10-31 c

Fig 10-31 (b, c) Panoramic X-ray and lateral cephalograph showing limited height at the posterior maxilla.

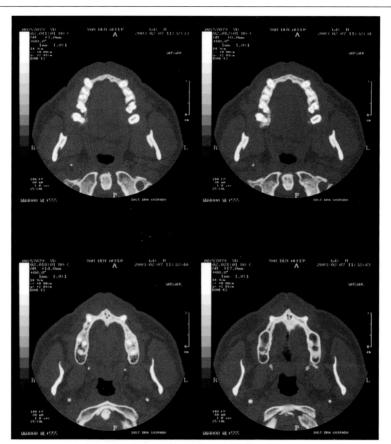

Fig 10-31 d

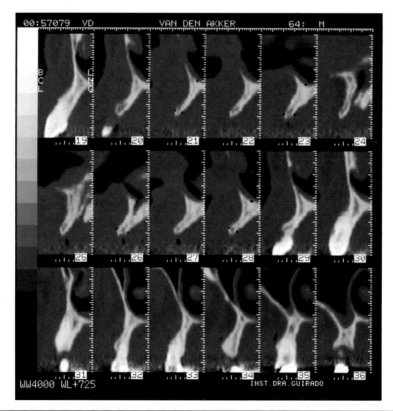

Fig 10-31 e

Fig 10-31 (d, e) CT scan depicting severe AP atrophy in the anterior maxilla.

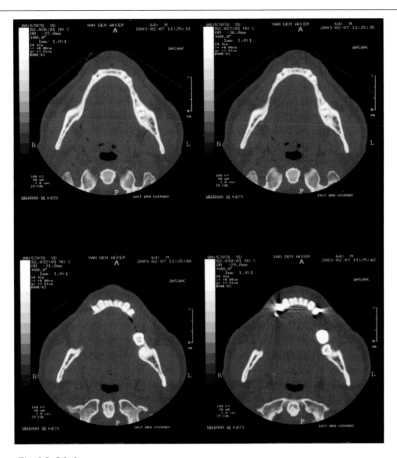

Fig 10-31 f

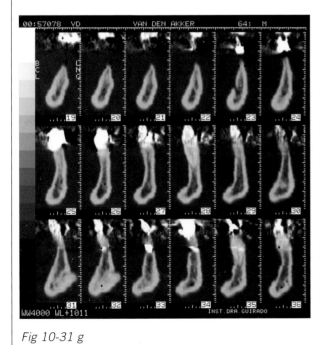

Fig 10-31 g

Fig 10-31 h

Fig 10-31 (f-h) Situation at the posterior mandible bilaterally. After evaluation of clinical and radiological information, full reconstruction with corticocancellous blocks is planned.

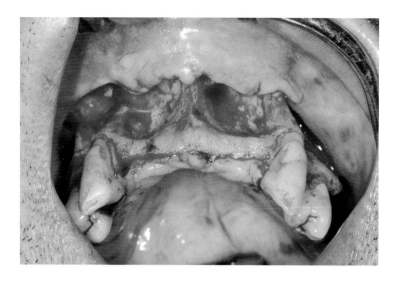

Fig 10-31 (i) De-globing of the anterior maxilla confirms the CT data. Disuse atrophy has narrowed the crest.

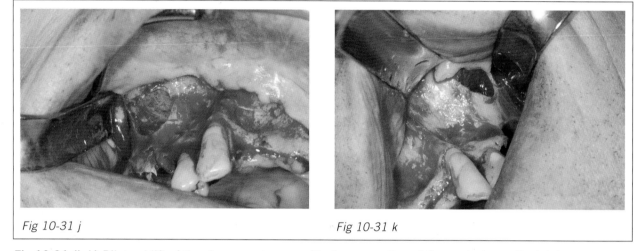

Fig 10-31 j

Fig 10-31 k

Fig 10-31 (j, k) Bilateral lift of the sinus membranes will allow correction of the posterior vertical defects.

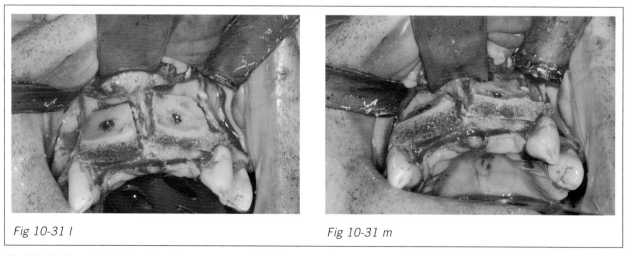

Fig 10-31 l

Fig 10-31 m

Fig 10-31 (l, m) Anterior ridge is reconstructed with two corticocancellous blocks. Note how the cancellous part of the veneers faces the defect. Vascular in-growth from the recipient site is easier into the medullary side of the graft.

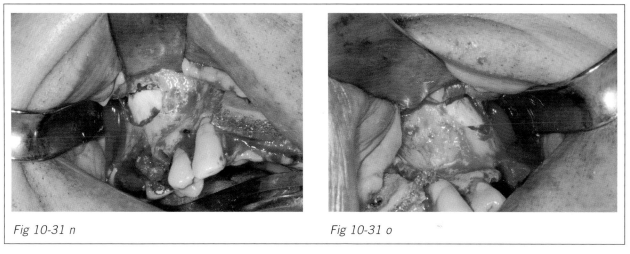

Fig 10-31 n

Fig 10-31 o

Fig 10-31 (n, o) Extra cancellous bone is used to fill both sinuses.

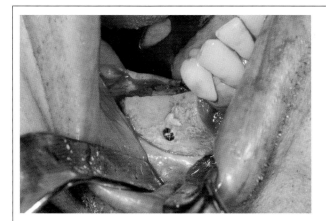

Fig 10-31 p

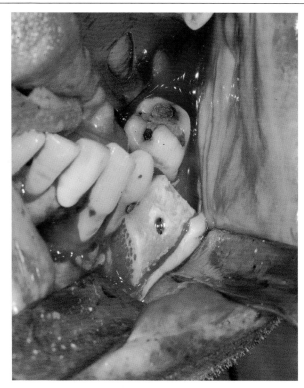

Fig 10-31 (p, q) Two additional blocks are fixed in a veneer fashion to correct width deficiency at posterior mandibular ridges. Note how, irrespective of the graft size, a single compression screw is sufficient.

Fig 10-31 q

187

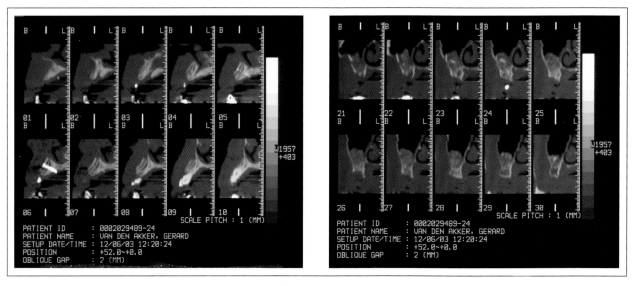

Fig 10-31 (r) Radiographic control post-reconstruction.

188

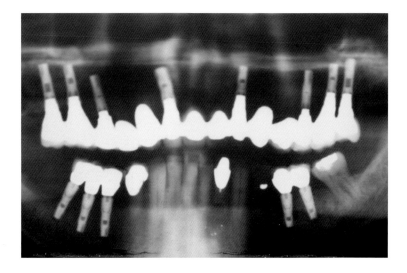

Fig 10-31 (s) Final result.

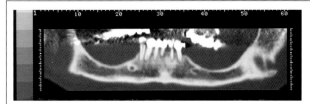

Fig 10-32 a

Fig 10-32 (a, b) This case presented with severe vertical atrophy in the posterior maxilla and mandible as well as a narrow ridge at the upper premolars.

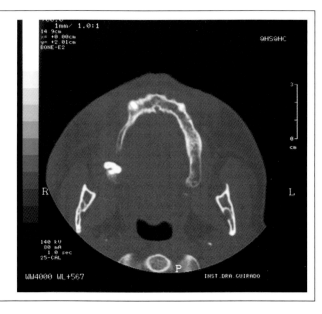

Fig 10-32 b

Fig 10-32 (c) Maxillo-mandibular reconstruction of all the defective zones is planned. Corticocancellous blocks are harvested and trimmed to on-lay graft the posterior mandibular areas. Note how one compression screw is stabilising the graft against the host site. These types of blocks have elastic properties, allowing bending and perfect adaptation to the recipient site. Note how the bundle exits the mental foramen.

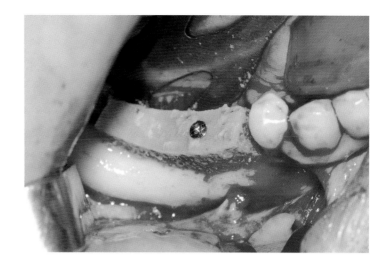

Fig 10-32 (d) It is essential to plan the positioning of the screws in order to avoid injury to the neurovascular bundle. On the right side, two blocks were tailored to reconstruct the defect.

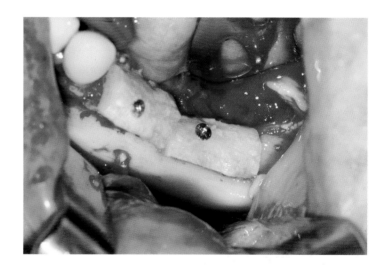

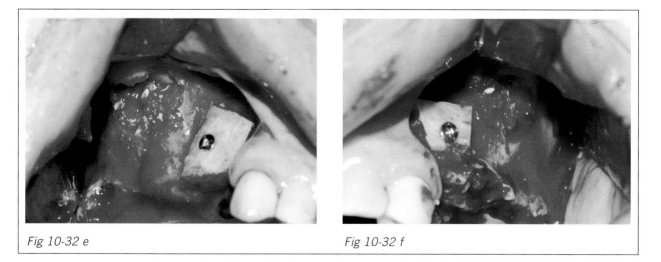

Fig 10-32 e   *Fig 10-32 f*

Fig 10-32 (e, f) Posterior maxilla was reconstructed by veneering the ridge in the premolar area and through a bilateral sinus lift.

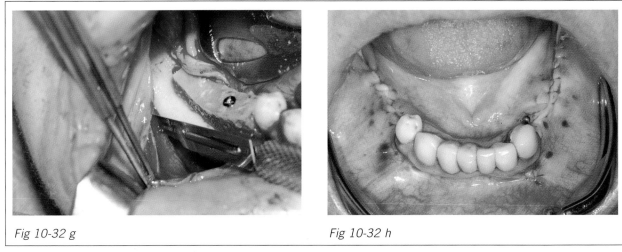

Fig 10-32 g

Fig 10-32 h

Fig 10-32 (g, h) Releasing incisions in the periosteum allow tensionless closure. Care must be taken when performing the releasing incisions to stay at the periosteal level, thus avoiding nerve branches.

Fig 10-32 i

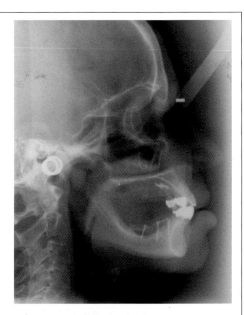

Fig 10-32 j

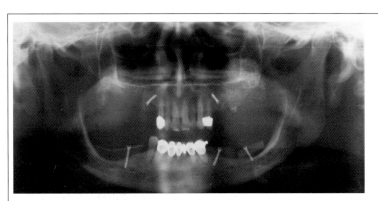

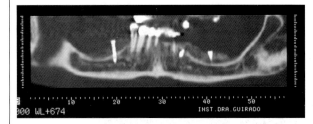

Fig 10-32 k

Fig 10-32 (i, l) Radiographic check three months after the reconstruction before implant placement.

Fig 10-32 l

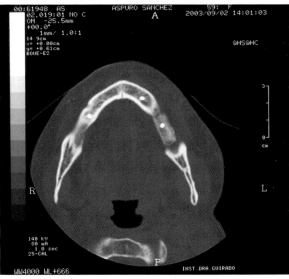

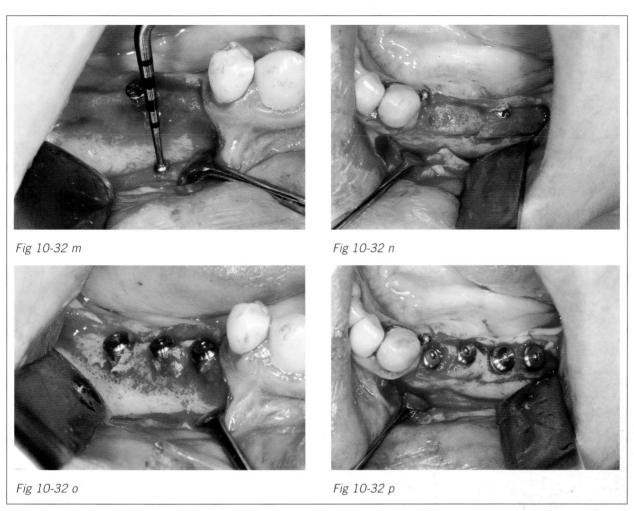

Fig 10-32 m

Fig 10-32 n

Fig 10-32 o

Fig 10-32 p

Fig 10-32 (m-p) Vertical increase in the posterior mandibular areas allows placement of 9mm fixtures. Remodelling and slight resorption has already started. When blocks from the IC are used we recommend not waiting more than three months before fixture placement.

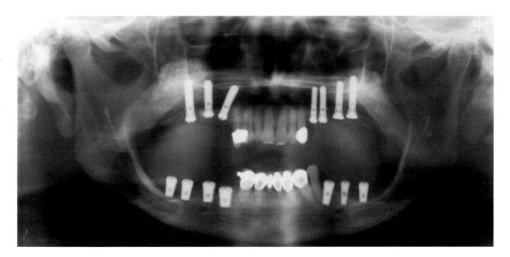

Fig 10-32 (q) Panoramic X-ray after fixture placement.

191

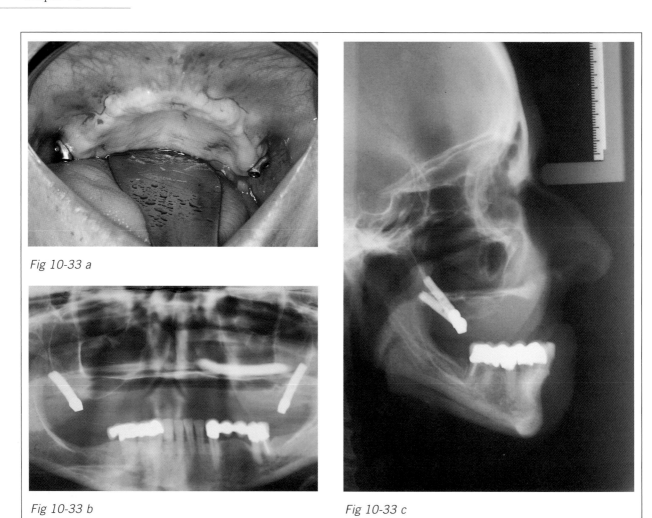

Fig 10-33 a

Fig 10-33 b

Fig 10-33 c

Fig 10-33 (a-c) Patient with total maxillary atrophy for which correction was attempted by placing implants in the paranasal and pterygoid buttresses. The former failed, and a plan was proposed to reconstruct the maxilla and at the same time correct sagital and vertical relationships.

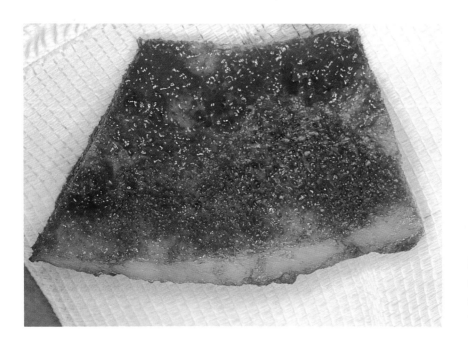

Fig 10-33 (d) Working with two surgical teams simultaneously saves surgical time. A block from the anterior IC was harvested.

Fig 10-33 (e, f) Access to the atrophic maxilla is achieved via a high sublabial incision. Submucosal dissection is carried out until the level of the osteotomy is reached. Then dissection proceeds in a subperiosteal fashion. Limited periosteal elevation warrants adequate vascular supply to the atrophic maxilla.

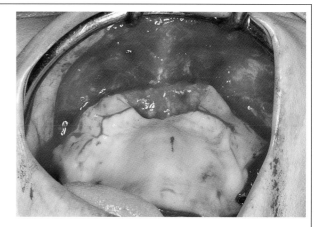

Fig 10-33 e

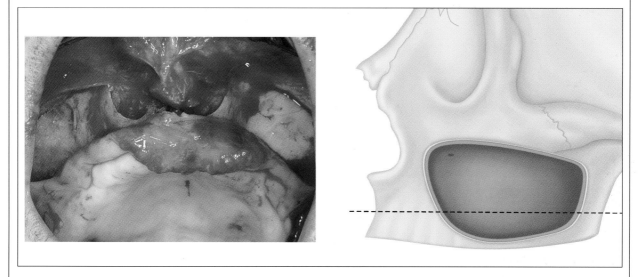

Fig 10-33 f

193

Fig 10-33 (g) A modified Le Fort I osteotomy is completed to avoid posteriorly the already positioned and perfectly integrated pterygoid fixtures. Downfracture of the maxilla has to be undertaken with care in order not to create undesired fractures within the mobilised and extremely atrophic maxilla.

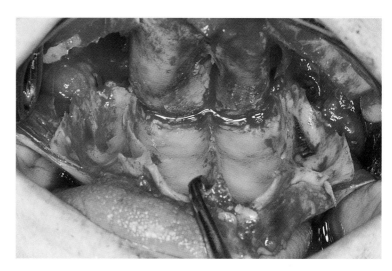

Fig 10-33 h

Fig 10-33 i

Fig 10-33 (h, i) Posteriorly, the anterior palatine arteries are identified in a crest located between the floor of the nose and maxillary sinus on each side.

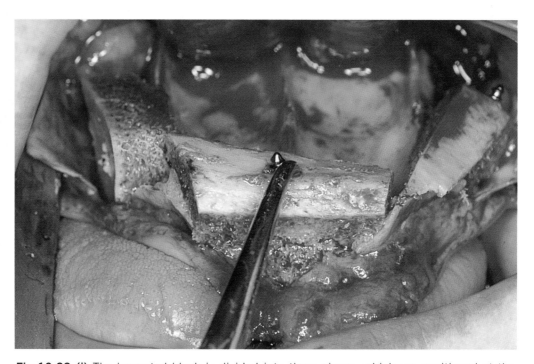

Fig 10-33 (j) The harvested block is divided into three pieces, which are positioned at the anterior nasal floor and floor of sinuses respectively. Blocks are fixed in place with bicortical screws.

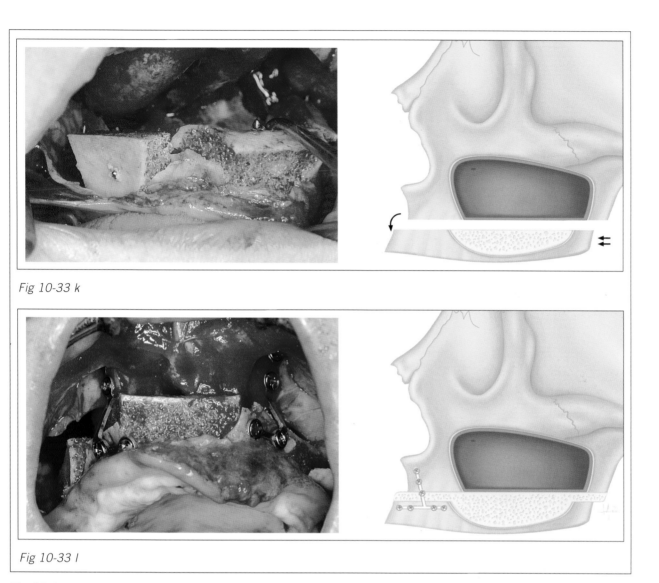

Fig 10-33 k

Fig 10-33 l

Fig 10-33 (k, l) Once reconstructed with interpositional grafts, the maxilla is repositioned both sagitally and vertically to normalise the tri-dimensional relationship with the mandible and the rest of the face. The newly repositioned maxilla is stabilised in place with plates and screws.

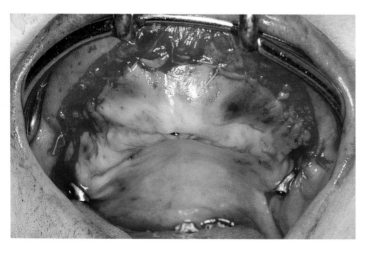

Fig 10-33 (m) A modified vestibuloplasty allows watertight closure of the reconstruction, still maintaining adequate depth of the vestibule. This will allow the patient to wear a removable denture one week postoperatively. The raw area heals secondarily with mucosal metaplasia.

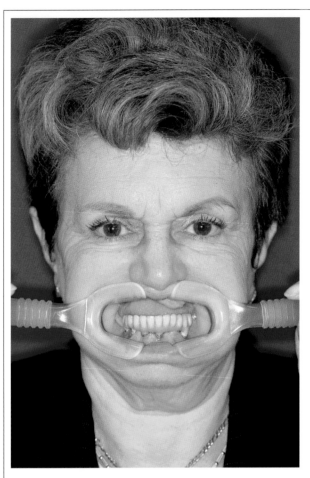

Fig 10-34 a

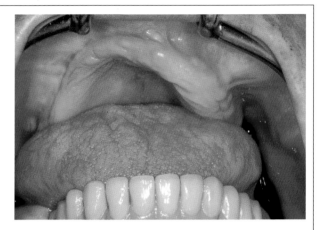

Fig 10-34 b

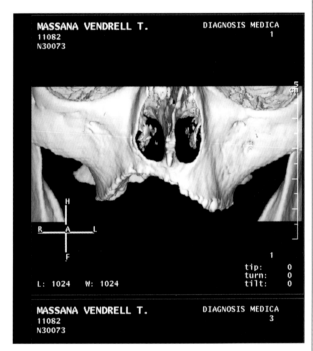

Fig 10-34 c

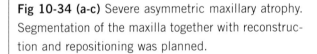
Fig 10-34 (a-c) Severe asymmetric maxillary atrophy. Segmentation of the maxilla together with reconstruction and repositioning was planned.

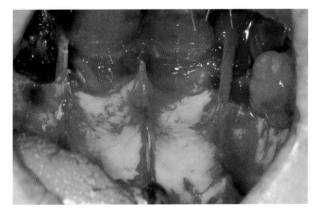

Fig 10-34 (d) Downfracturing of the maxilla is followed by pedicle identification.

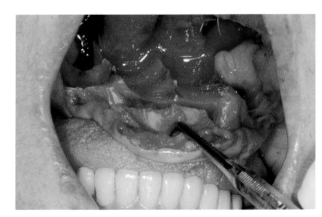

Fig 10-34 (e) Segmentation of the maxilla is done in order to achieve symmetry.

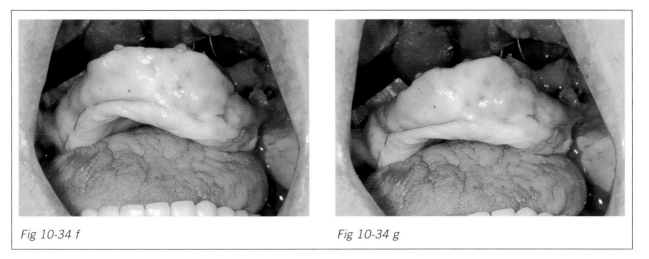

Fig 10-34 f

Fig 10-34 g

Fig 10-34 (f, g) Segmentation allows correction of the upper occlusal plane.

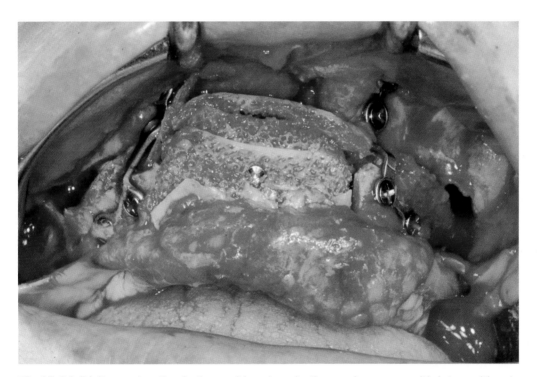

Fig 10-34 (h) Reconstruction is then achieved, as in the previous case, with interpositional blocks from the IC. Once reconstructed to a normal volume, the maxilla is repositioned and fixed with plates and screws.

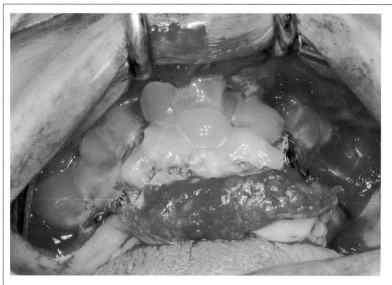

Fig 10-34 i

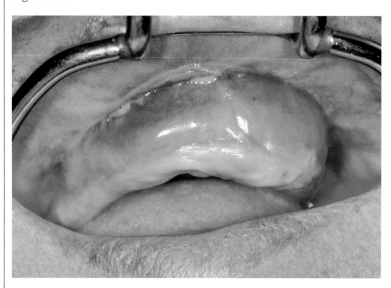

Fig 10-34 j

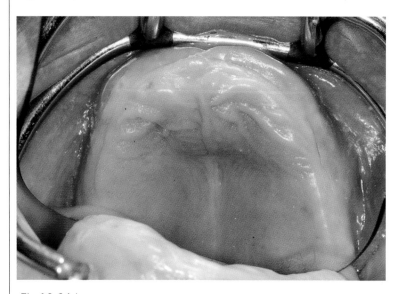

Fig 10-34 k

Fig 10-34 (i-k) PRP is used to protect the reconstruction, and a modified vestibuloplasty allows the use of a complete removable denture 10 days after the procedure. Note normalisation of shape and symmetry.

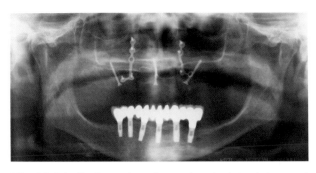

Fig 10-34 (l) Control radiographs depict plates and screws used in the procedure. 18mm screws were used for graft stabilisation.

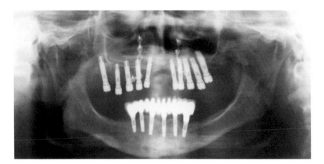

Fig 10-34 (m) Two months after the procedure, 10 fixtures were placed. At the same time all the screws located in the area of implant insertion were removed. The plates and upper screws are left in place to avoid excessive de-globing of the middle third of the face.

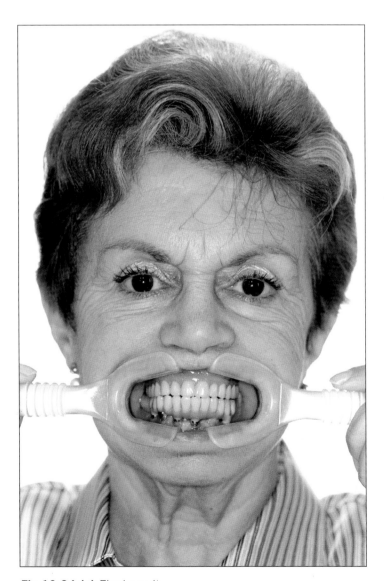

Fig 10-34 (n) Final result.

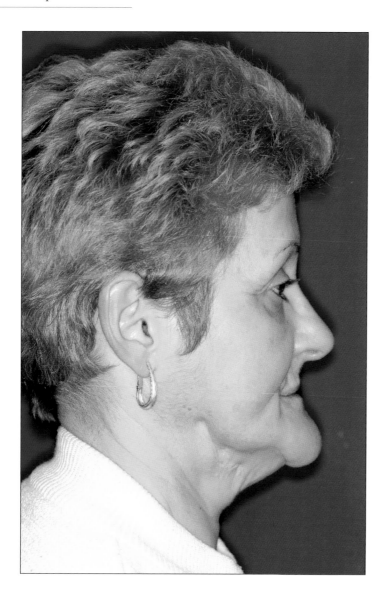

Fig 10-35 (a) Total maxillo-mandibular atrophy secondary to long-standing edentulism and use of removable dentures. Lateral picture of the patient is with dentures in place.

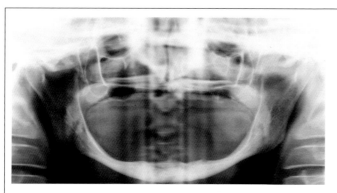

Fig 10-35 b

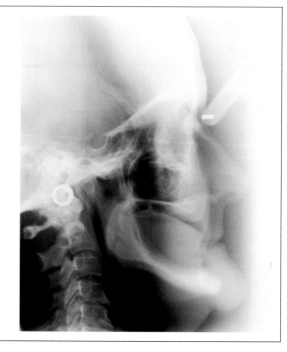

Fig 10-35 (b, c) Standard radiographs show the degree of atrophy.

Fig 10-35 c

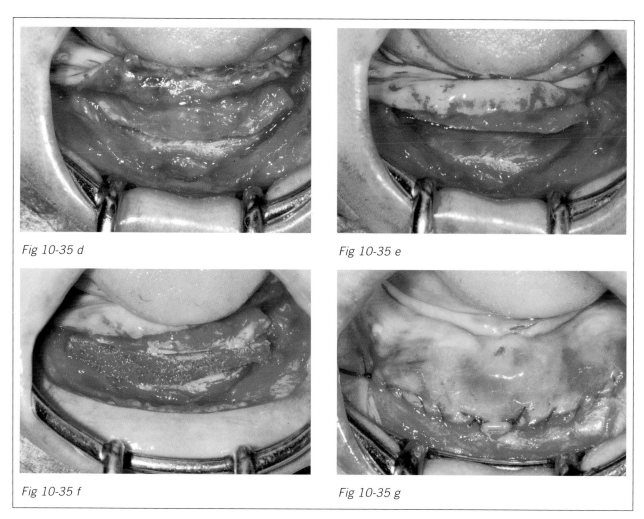

Fig 10-35 d

Fig 10-35 e

Fig 10-35 f

Fig 10-35 g

Fig 10-35 (d-g) A 'sandwich' procedure is undertaken in the mandible interposing a block from the IC. Tricortical stabilisation is achieved with a single 18mm compression screw.

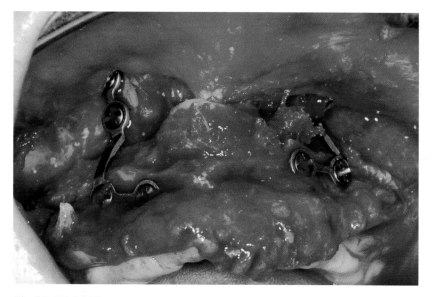

Fig 10-35 (h) The same procedure is completed in the maxilla, as described in the previous two cases.

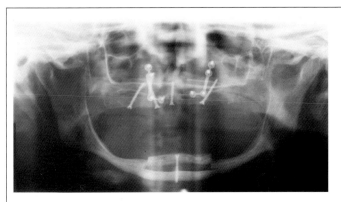

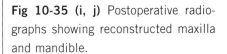

Fig 10-35 i

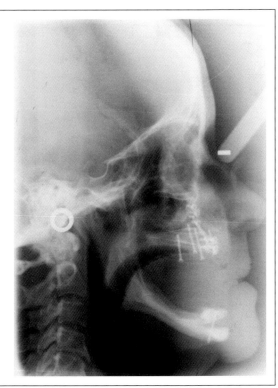

Fig 10-35 (i, j) Postoperative radiographs showing reconstructed maxilla and mandible.

Fig 10-35 j

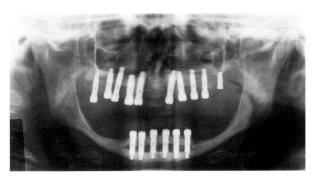

Fig 10-35 (k) Fixtures placed two months after the main procedure.

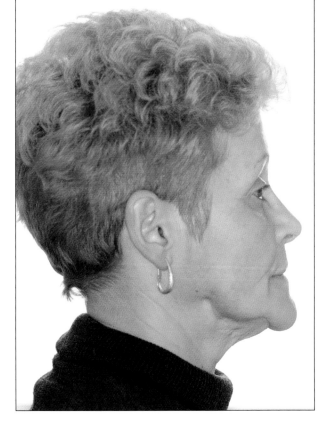

Fig 10-35 (l) Final result. Note transformation of the face from short and concave to long and convex.

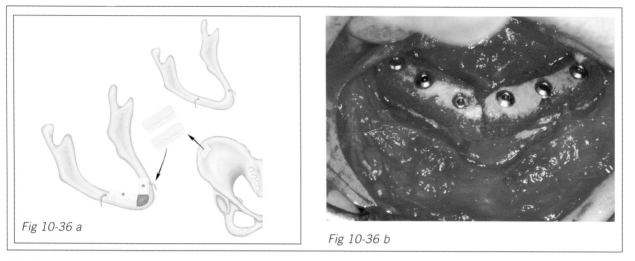

Fig 10-36 a

Fig 10-36 b

Fig 10-36 (a, b) Corticocancellous blocks from the iliac crest are useful for reconstruction in severe mandibular atrophy. The grafts can be fixed by the implants.

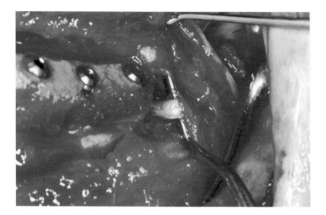

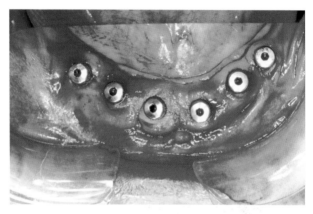

Fig 10-36 (c) Care should be taken to adapt the grafts so the mental nerves are not disturbed.

Fig 10-36 (d) Abutment connection five months after reconstruction. The fact that both grafts and fixtures are placed at one stage shortens the treatment time, thus minimising graft resorption.

203

Minimally invasive bone harvest with trephines

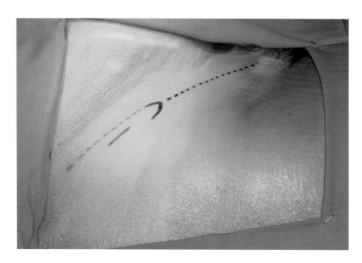

Fig 10-37 (a) Reference marks over the crest. Note position of anterosuperior spine.

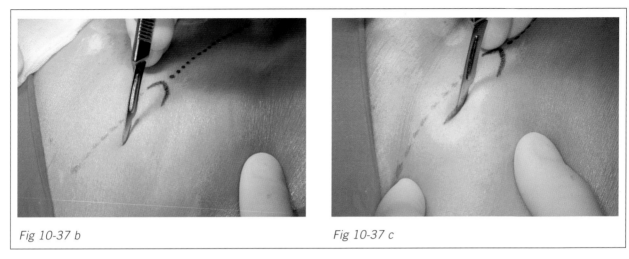

Fig 10-37 b

Fig 10-37 c

Fig 10-37 (b, c) A No.10 or No.15 scalpel is used to produce a 10mm stab incision directly over the crest.

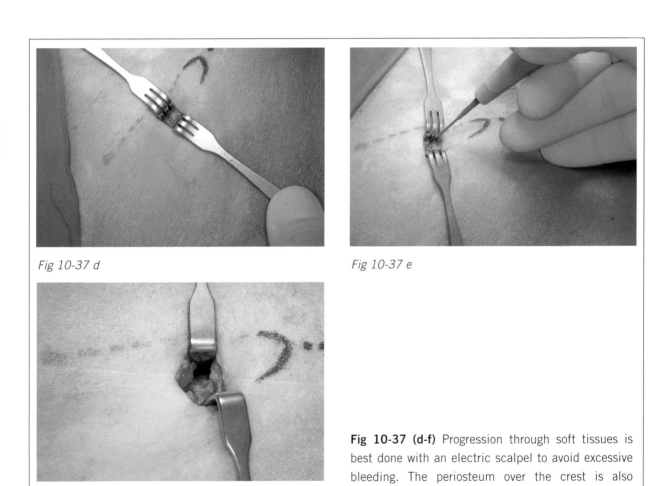

Fig 10-37 d

Fig 10-37 e

Fig 10-37 f

Fig 10-37 (d-f) Progression through soft tissues is best done with an electric scalpel to avoid excessive bleeding. The periosteum over the crest is also incised.

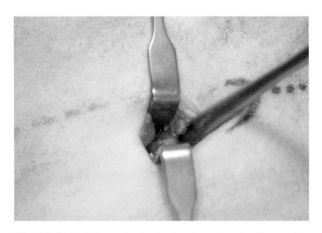

Fig 10-37 (g) A periosteal elevator retracts the perio-steum sufficiently to facilitate access with the trephine.

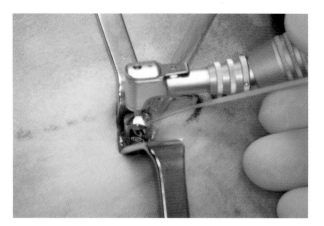

Fig 10-37 (h) An 8mm trephine opens a bony window in the crest, wide enough to place a bone curette.

Fig 10-37 (i) The bone curette is used to free the can-cellous bone within the iliac crest.

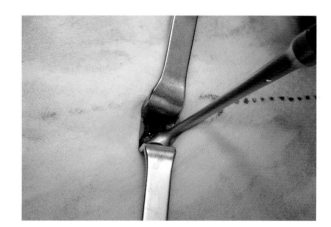

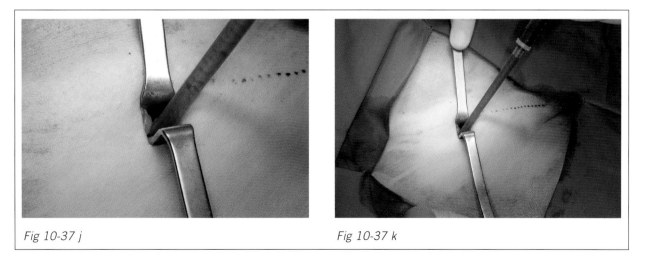

Fig 10-37 j

Fig 10-37 k

Fig 10-37 (j, k) As in the tibia technique, a bone filter is used to collect the released bone.

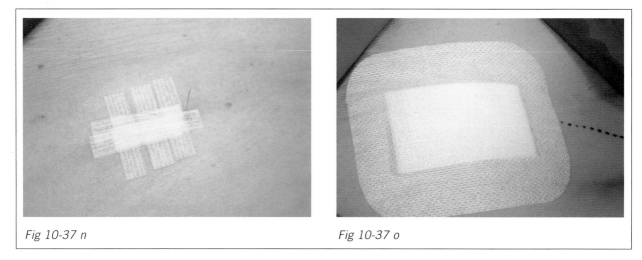

Fig 10-37 l

Fig 10-37 m

Fig 10-37 (l, m) A deep resorbable plane is completed with 4/0 suture and a subcuticular plane with 5/0 nylon. The latter will be removed in seven days.

Fig 10-37 n

Fig 10-37 o

Fig 10-37 (n, o) A small dressing is placed to protect the area from clothing.

References

1 Cordeiro PG, Santamaria E, Kraus DH, et al. Reconstruction of total maxillectomy defects with preservation of the orbital contents. Plast Reconstr Surg 1998;102:1874-1887.

2 Pogrel MA, Podlesh S, Anthony JP, Alexander J. A comparison of vascularized and nonvascularized bone grafts for reconstruction of mandibular continuity defects. J Oral Maxillofac Surg 1997;55:1200-1206.

3 Swart JG, Allard RH. Subperiosteal onlay augmentation of the mandible: A clinical and radiographic survey. J Oral Maxillofac Surg 198;43:183-187.

4 Fazili M, van der Dussen FM, van Waas MA. Long-term results of augmentation of the atrophic mandible. Int J Oral Maxillofac Surg 1986;15:513-520.

5 Sailer HF. A new method of inserting endosseous implants in totally atrophic maxillae. J Craniomaxillofac Surg 1989;17:299-305.

6 Isaksson S, Ekfeldt A, Alberius P, Blomqvist JE. Early results from reconstruction of severely atrophic (Class VI) maxillas by immediate endosseous implants in conjunction with bone grafting and Le Fort I osteotomy. Int J Oral Maxillofac Surg 1993;22:144-148.

7 Misch CE, Dietsh F. Endosteal implants and iliac crest grafts to restore severely resorbed totally edentulous maxillae: A retrospective study. J Oral Implantol 1994;20:100-110.

8 Collins M, James DR, Mars M. Alveolar bone grafting: A review of 115 patients. Eur J Orthod 1998;20:115-120.

9 Misch CE, Dietsh F. Autogenous bone grafts for endosteal implants: Indications and failures. Int J Oral Implantol 1991;8:13-20.

10 Ilankovan V, Stronczek M, Telfer M, et al. A prospective study of trephined bone grafts of the tibial shaft and iliac crest. Br J Oral Maxillofac Surg 1998;36:434-439.

11 Ebraheim NA, Yang H, Lu J, et al. Anterior iliac crest bone graft: Anatomic considerations. Spine 1997;22: 847-849.

12 Mazock JB, Schow SR, Triplett RG. Posterior iliac crest bone harvest: Review of technique, complications, and use of an epidural catheter for postoperative pain control. J Oral Maxillofac Surg 2003;61:1497-1503.

13 De la Torre JI, Tenenhaus M, Gallagher PM, Sachs SA. Harvesting iliac bone graft: Decreasing the morbidity. Cleft Palate Craniofac J 1999;36:388-390.

14 Caminiti MF, Sandor GK, Carmichael RP. Quantification of bone harvested from the iliac crest using a power-driven trephine. J Oral Maxillofac Surg 1999;57:801-806.

15 Sandor GK, Rittenberg BN, Clokie CM, Caminiti MF. Clinical success in harvesting autogenous bone using a minimally invasive trephine. J Oral Maxillofac Surg 2003;61:164-168.

16 Sherman R, Chapman WC, Hannon G, Block JE. Control of bone bleeding at the sternum and iliac crest donor sites using a collagen-based composite combined with autologous plasma: Results of a randomized controlled trial. Orthopedics 2001;24:137-141.

17 Sasso RC, Williams JI, Dimasi N, Meyer PR Jr. Postoperative drains at the donor sites of iliac-crest bone grafts: A prospective, randomized study of morbidity at the donor site in patients who had a traumatic injury of the spine. J Bone Joint Surg Am 1998;80:631-635.

18 Hoard MA, Bill TJ, Campbell RL. Reduction in morbidity after iliac crest bone harvesting: The concept of preemptive analgesia. J Craniofac Surg 1998;9:448-451.

19 Gundes H, Kilickan L, Gurkan Y, et al. Short- and long-term effects of regional application of morphine and bupivacaine on the iliac crest donor site. Acta Orthop Belg. 2000;66:341-344.

20 Hurzeler MB, Kirsch A, Ackermann KL, Quinones CR. Reconstruction of the severely resorbed maxilla with dental implants in the augmented maxillary sinus: A 5-year clinical investigation. Int J Oral Maxillofac Implants 1996;11:466-475.

21 Kahnberg KE, Nilsson P, Rasmusson L. Le Fort I osteotomy with interpositional bone grafts and implants for rehabilitation of the severely resorbed maxilla: A 2-stage procedure. Int J Oral Maxillofac Implants 1999;14:571-578.

22 Neyt LF, De Clercq CA, Abeloos JV, Mommaerts MY. Reconstruction of the severely resorbed maxilla with a combination of sinus augmentation, onlay bone grafting, and implants. J Oral Maxillofac Surg 1997;55:1397-1401

23 Chiapasco M, Abati S, Romeo E, Vogel G. Clinical outcome of autogenous bone blocks or guided bone regeneration with e-PTFE membranes for the reconstruction of narrow edentulous ridges. Clin Oral Implants Res 1999; 10:278-288.

24 Kalk WW, Raghoebar GM, Jansma J, Boering G. Morbidity from iliac crest bone harvesting. J Oral Maxillofac Surg 1996;54:1424-1430.

25 Acocella A, Nardi P, Tedesco A, et al. Anterior iliac bone grafts: Techniques and sequelae. Report on 107 cases and review of the literature. Minerva Stomatol 2003;52: 441-453.

26 Mirovsky Y, Neuwirth M. Injuries to the lateral femoral cutaneous nerve during spine surgery. Spine 2000;25: 1266-1269.

27 Nocini PF, Bedogni A, Valsecchi S, et al. Fractures of the iliac crest following anterior and posterior bone graft harvesting: Review of the literature and case presentation. Minerva Stomatol 2003;52:441-452.

28 Heary RF, Schlenk RP, Sacchieri TA, et al. Persistent iliac crest donor site pain: Independent outcome assessment. Neurosurgery 2002;50:510-517.

29 Porras M, Lindahl J, Saarinen O. Retroperitoneal haemorrhage after taking bone graft from the anterior iliac crest: Report of two cases. J Trauma 2003;55:141-143.

30 Danikas D, Theodorou SJ, Stratoulias C, et al. Hernia through an iliac crest bone-graft donor site. Plast Reconstr Surg 2002;110:1612-1613.

11

Tibia

Previous studies have pointed out the advantages of using the proximal tibia as a donor site when large amounts of cancellous bone are needed.[1-6] Tibial bone harvesting has less morbidity than iliac crest bone harvesting.[6] Iliac crest grafting requires general anaesthesia in most instances. Higher quantities of cancellous bone can be harvested from the tibia than from anterior or posterior iliac crest.

Tibial bone harvesting for reconstruction in oral surgery has been advocated by several authors,[7,8] and several studies have compared complication rates and amount of bone harvested with this technique with that of iliac crest harvesting.[6] Conclusions of these studies favour tibial bone harvesting in cases were high amounts of cancellous bone are needed.

Different approaches and methods for recruiting bone from the proximal tibia have been proposed,[1-7] with variable results regarding amount of bone and postoperative disturbances.

Some authors advocate the use of the so-called 'lateral approach'.[2] The claim is that higher amounts can be harvested this way. However, it has been recently proven that similar amounts of bone can be harvested from both approaches.[8]

Depending on the authors, 10-42cc of cancellous bone can be harvested.[1-8] In our series, a mean of 28cc was obtained.

Surgical Anatomy

The proximal end of the tibia is expanded transversely. This end has medial and lateral condyles, an intercondylar area and the tibial tuberosity. The anterior condylar surfaces are continuous, with a large triangular area, the apex of which is distal and formed by the tibial tuberosity. This is divided into a rough distal and a smooth proximal region (Fig 11-1). The former can be easily palpated and is separated from the skin by a subcutaneous infrapatellar bursa. The ligamentum patellae is attached to the proximal region.[1]

A major portion of the tibia is subcutaneous and, at its cephalad extent, the tibial condyles can be palpated immediately below the knee.

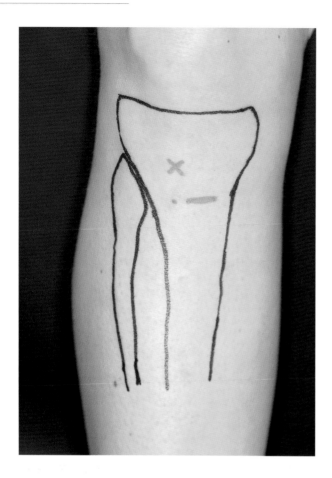

Fig 11-1 The proximal end of the tibia is an excellent source of cancellous bone.

On the anterior surface of the proximal end of the tibia between the condyles the tibial tuberosity can be palpated as an oval protuberance. Palpation of this tubercle is essential to avoid violation of the articular surface of the tibial plateau and damage to the knee joint.[2]

Small blood vessels in the immediate vicinity of the lateral proximal tibia include branches of the medial superior and inferior genicular arteries passing under cover of the patellar ligament; branches of the medial superior and inferior genicular arteries passing under cover of the patellar ligament; branches of the lateral inferior, genicular, fibular and the anterior recurrent tibial; and branches of the anterior tibial arteries.

The tibialis anterior muscle is located on the lateral surface of the tibia and in the caudal extent of the dissection is thick and fleshy. Its fibres course vertically caudal, overlapping the anterior tibial vessels and deep peroneal nerve in the proximal tibial region.

A line across the tuberosity signals the distal limit of the epiphyseal line. The shaft is triangular and has medial, lateral and posterior surfaces. The lateral surface is between the anterior and interosseous borders, and the proximal three quarters is attached to the tibialis anterior muscle. The tibia is ossified from three distinct centres, the shaft and both epiphyses. The proximal epiphyseal centre is usually present at birth and at about 10 years of age a thin anterior process descends to form the smooth part of the tibial tuberosity.[3]

Surgical Procedure

For procurement of the tibial graft, we have developed an original technique of cancellous bone harvesting from the proximal tibia through a medial approach.

Anaesthesia

Mild intravenous sedation, consisting of meperidine and methoxital, is administered. Surgical field isolation is achieved through sterile drapes after scrub decontamination with iodine.

A 10mm horizontal line following skin creases is drawn 20mm below and 20mm medially from the anterior tibial tuberosity (Fig 11-2). Lidocaine (2%) with epinephrine (1:80.000) is then infiltrated subcutaneously and at the level of the periosteum.

Access

A through-and-through incision, skin to bone, is made with a 10 blade (Fig 11-3).

Lateral reflection of the periosteum is completed with a sharp periosteal elevator in order to expose enough bone surface for the trephine access.

Harvesting procedure

A manual trephine 8mm in diameter is used to remove a tape of bone of the same size (Fig 11-4 a-b). With the assistance of different sizes of straight and angled bone curettes, cancellous bone is mobilised within the proximal compartment of the tibia (Fig 11-5 a-c). No attempt is made to pull the bone out of the tibia with the curettes since they act only as scrappers to loosen the cancellous bone from the cortical walls within the compartment.

211

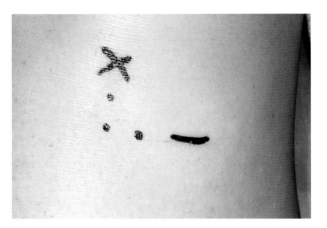

Fig 11-2 References to be considered are: 20mm under and 20mm medial to anterior tibialis tuberosity.

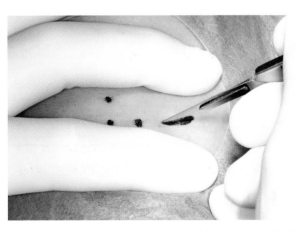

Fig 11-3 Through-and-through incision with a No.10 blade, on a skin crease and passing directly to the bone.

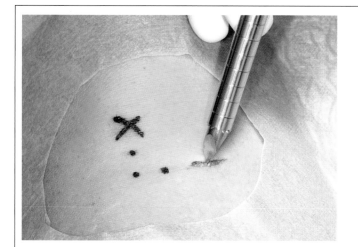

Fig 11-4 a

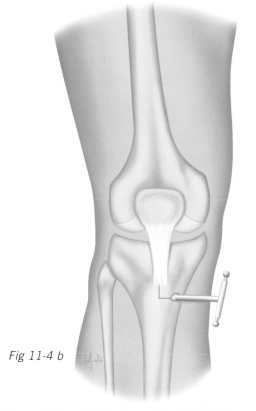

Fig 11-4 (a, b) A trephine 8mm in diameter is manually inserted to open a round bony window.

Fig 11-4 b

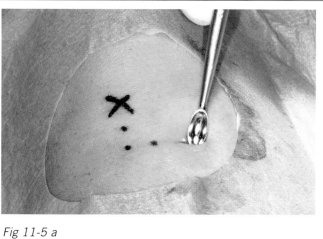

Fig 11-5 b

Fig 11-5 a

Fig 11-5 (a-c) A curette inserted through the window helps in loosening the cancellous bone.

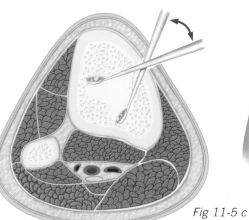

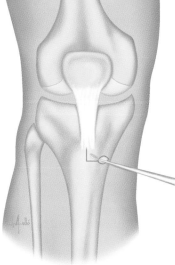

Fig 11-5 c

A bone aspirator with a filter (Bone-trap, Astra, Malmo, Sweden) is used to collect the loose bone (Fig 11-6 a-d). This sequence is repeated as many times as needed until the cortical walls of the proximal tibia are peeled off cancellous bone. When no further bone is trapped into the bone filter the compartment is filled up with saline injected under pressure. Then a final filter aspiration of the cavity allows for further gathering of bone remnants.

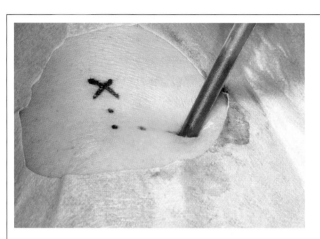

Fig 11-6 a

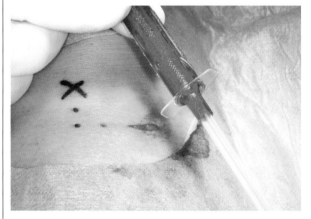

Fig 11-6 b

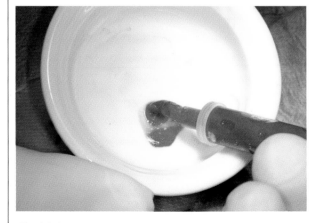

Fig 11-6 c

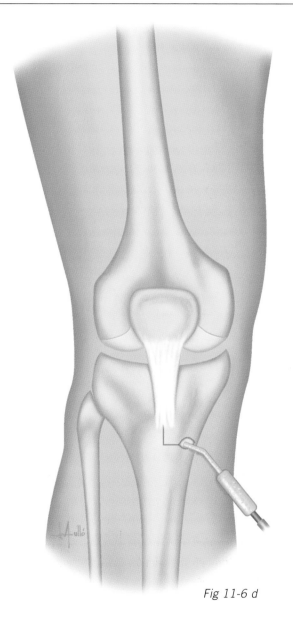

Fig 11-6 d

Fig 11-6 (a-d) A bone filter connected to suction is inserted through the hole to capture and remove the bone.

Finally, closing of the wound is made in three layers - periosteal, subcutaneous and subcuticular, the first two with interrupted 4/0 poliglactin sutures, the last with running 4/0 nylon (Fig 11-7).

Collected bone cores are kept in a porcelain dish and eventually mixed with PRP (Fig 11-8).

Postoperative care

An elastic dressing is applied incorporating knee, calf and ankle. Patients are sent home accompanied directly after the procedure. The bandage is removed after the first week, together with the subcuticular suture.

All patients are placed on antibiotics and NSAID for seven days.

Patients are instructed to avoid impact-loading of the operated leg for the first two months.

Complications

The medial approach to the proximal tibia has proven as effective as the lateral approach in terms of the amount of bone collected [8] and is also safer, avoiding potential injury to important structures. The limited access prevents weakening of the proximal tibia, thus reducing the risk for pathologic fractures at this level (Fig 11-9a, b). The lateral approach involves entering the anterior compartment of the lower extremity, whereas the medial approach does not violate any of the four lower extremity compartments. The bone is closer to the skin in the medial approach. Only insertions of the semi-membranous muscle are to be avoided.

Clinical Applications

The main indication for the tibia as a donor site in preprosthetic bone grafting is filling of moderate to large cavities where the graft can be self-retentive (Fig 10-11 to Fig 11-16).

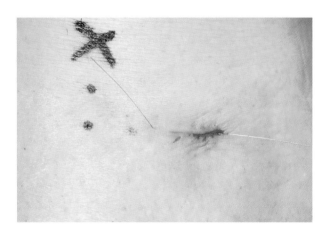

Fig 11-7 Periosteal suture is followed by a subcuticular 4/0 running suture.

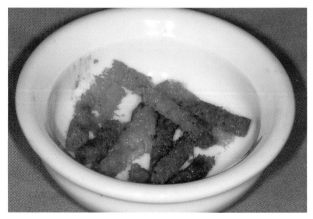

Fig 11-8 Collected bone.

214

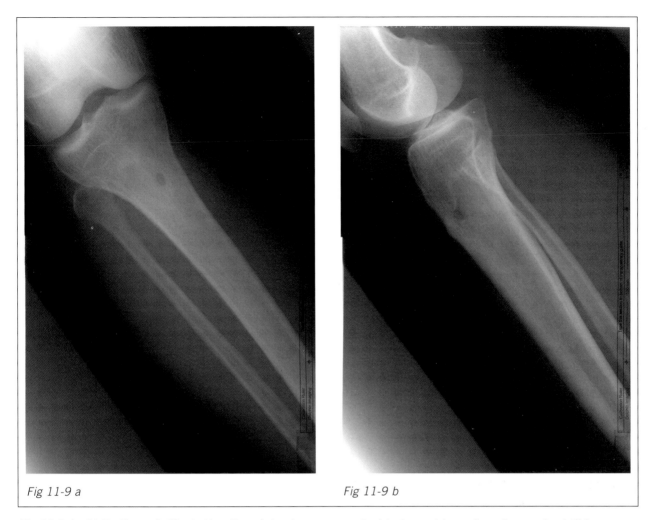

Fig 11-9 a   *Fig 11-9 b*

Fig 11-9 (a, b) Radiograph illustrating the minimal access required to harvest bone from the proximal tibia.

In the past two years, the tibia has become our site of choice for uni- or bilateral sinus grafting. The amount and quality of harvested bone enables predictable sinus reconstructions. The low morbidity associated with this technique has increased patient acceptance of reconstructive procedures. Except for those cases where bone blocks are needed (for instance, when wide disruption of the sinus membrane has occurred), we tend to favour the tibia as a donor site over the chin. The possibility of working simultaneously in two surgical fields, thus shortening operative time, makes this site very attractive.

Other indications for the tibia as a donor site are the filling of large cysts.

When mixed with PRP, cancellous bone can also be used for onlay bone grafting in transverse alveolar defects.

In cases where placement of implants will be delayed we recommend mixing of the autogenous bone with a bovine bone material to slow resorption.[9]

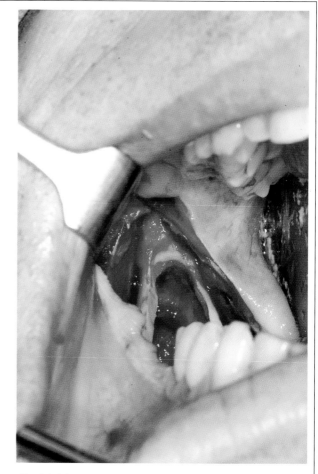

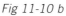

Fig 11-10 a

Fig 11-10 (a, b) Cylinders of medullary bone harvested to fill up a large cavity created in the posterior mandible after resecting a cyst.

Fig 11-10 b

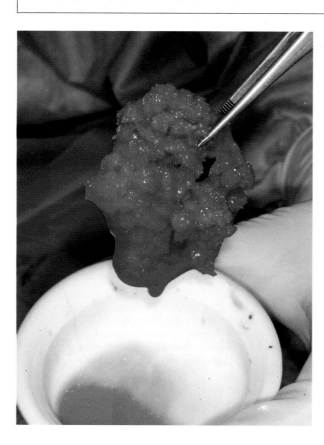

Fig 11-10 (c) Harvested bone is mixed with PRP to facilitate management of the graft.

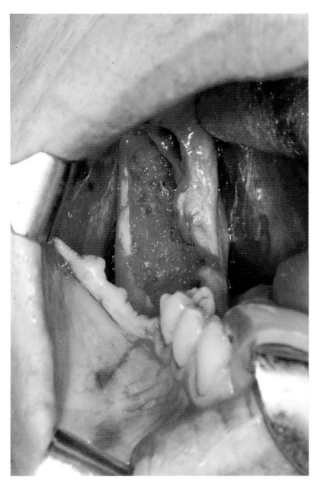

Fig 11-10 (d) Cavity filled with the mixture.

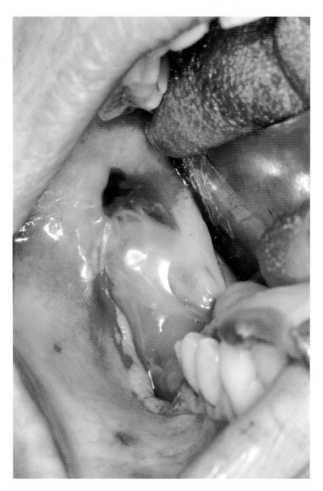

Fig 11-10 (e) Additional PRP helps in further protecting the reconstruction.

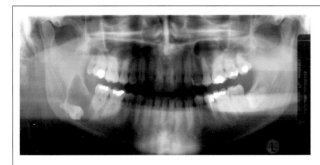

Fig 11-10 f

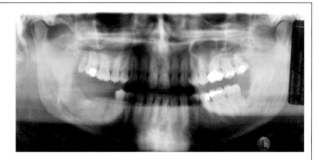

Fig 11-10 g

Fig 11-10 (f, g) Radiological images pre- and two months post-surgery. Note normalisation of bone density.

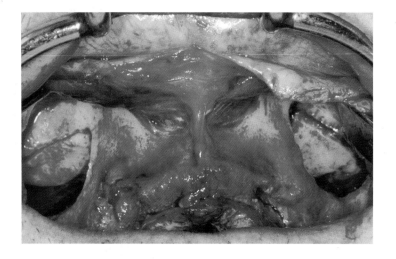

Fig 11-11 (a) Panoramic X-ray showing total edentulism in the upper jaw, with reduced available bone posteriorly due to hyperpneumatisation of the sinuses.

Fig 11-11 (b) Surgical access with bilateral lift of the sinus membrane.

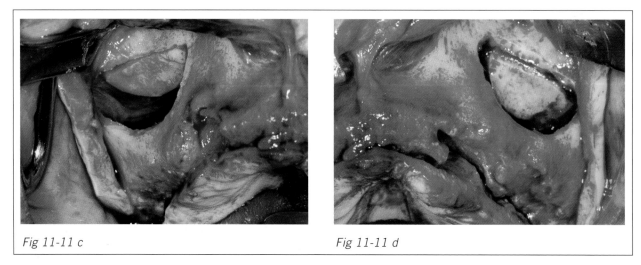

Fig 11-11 c

Fig 11-11 d

Fig 11-11 (c, d) Close-up of each side. Note the presence of bilateral crestal defects due to long-standing periodontal problems.

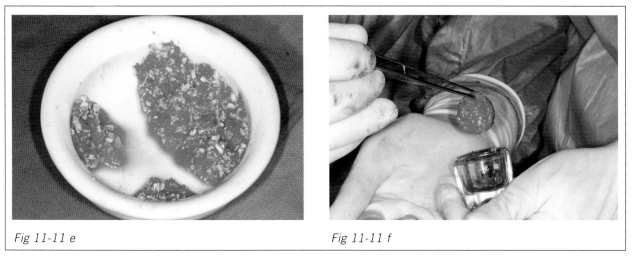

Fig 11-11 e

Fig 11-11 f

Fig 11-11 (e, f) Cancellous bone harvested from the tibia is mixed with PRP. A small (20%) percentage of anorganic bone substitute is added to delay resorption of the autogenous bone. We use this approach when implant placement is scheduled for a later stage, in order to preserve the graft until the fixtures are loaded. The anorganic matrix is also responsible for the radiological opacity during the first few months.

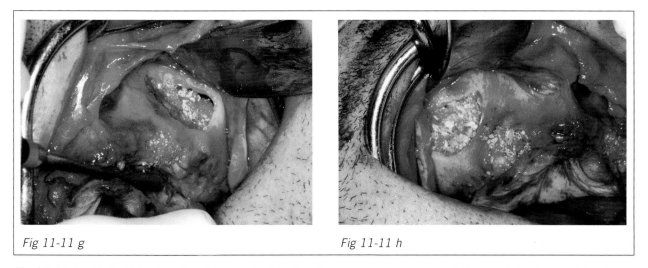

Fig 11-11 g

Fig 11-11 h

Fig 11-11 (g, h) Graft is placed and compacted in the sinus compartments and at the crestal defects bilaterally.

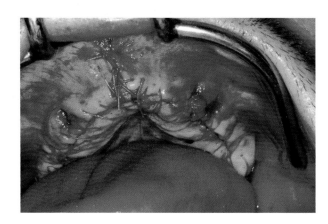

Fig 11-11 (i) As usual, a watertight suture is essential to protect the graft.

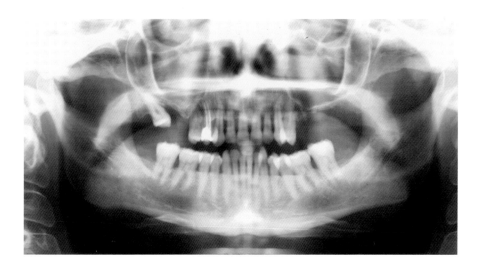

Fig 11-12 (a) Bilateral hyper-pneumatisation of the sinus. Bilateral sinus lift is planned with cancellous bone from the tibia.

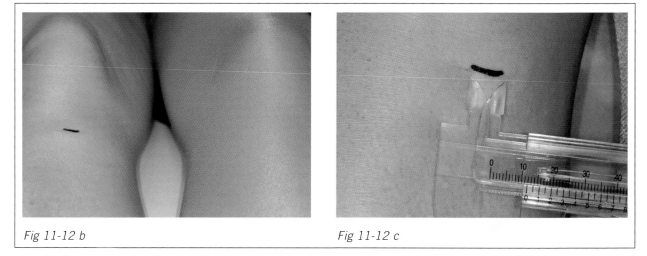

Fig 11-12 b

Fig 11-12 c

Fig 11-12 (b, c) Access line is drawn following anatomical references already mentioned.

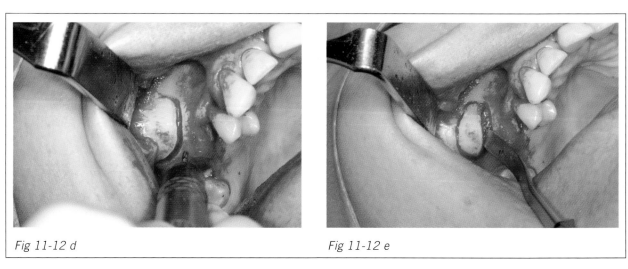

Fig 11-12 d

Fig 11-12 e

Fig 11-12 (d, e) Lateral access to the sinus with removal of the window.

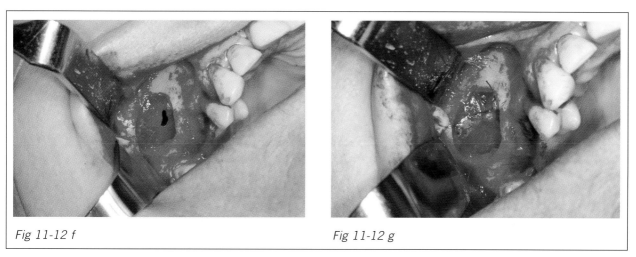

Fig 11-12 f

Fig 11-12 g

Fig 11-12 (f, g) A small tear in the membrane is detected and sutured.

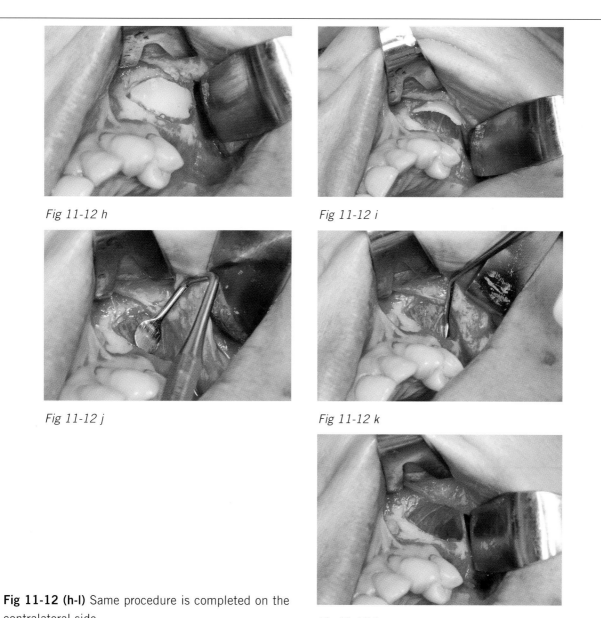

Fig 11-12 h

Fig 11-12 i

Fig 11-12 j

Fig 11-12 k

Fig 11-12 l

Fig 11-12 (h-l) Same procedure is completed on the contralateral side.

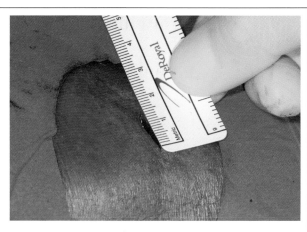

Fig 11-12 n

222

Fig 11-12 m

Fig 11-12 (m, n) Access to the tibia.

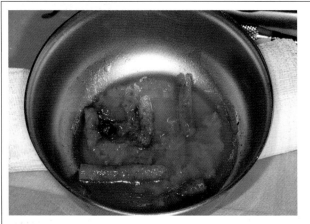

Fig 11-12 o

Fig 11-12 p

Fig 11-12 (o, p) Collected bone mixture is placed in two syringes in order to compress the graft and to facilitate placement in the sinuses.

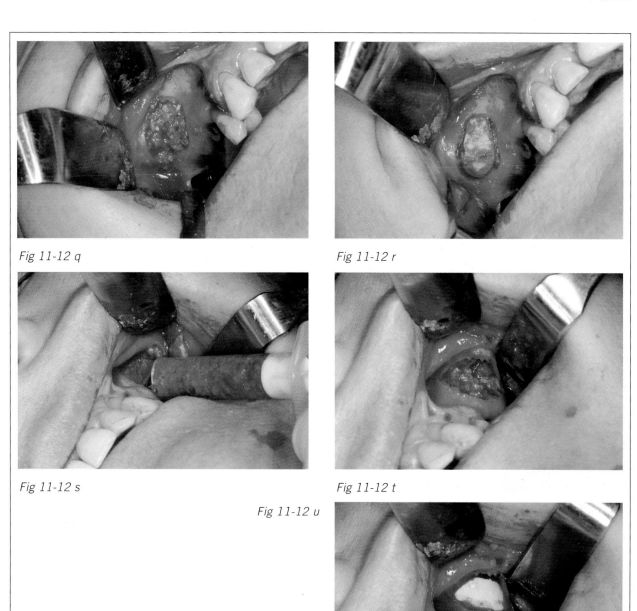

Fig 11-12 q

Fig 11-12 r

Fig 11-12 s

Fig 11-12 t

Fig 11-12 u

Fig 11-12 (q-u) Both sinuses are filled up with the compressed graft.

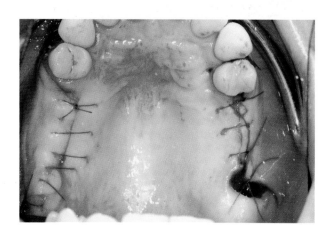

Fig 11-12 (v) Primary closure after removal of the remaining molar.

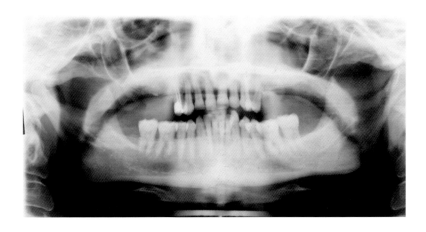

Fig 11-12 (x) Postoperative control showing increase of height at the posterior maxilla bilaterally.

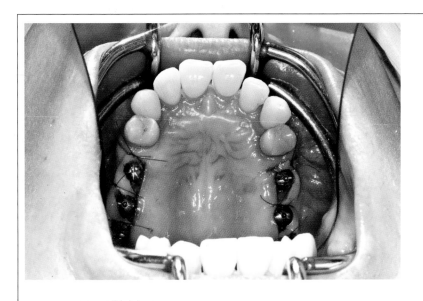

Fig 11-12 y

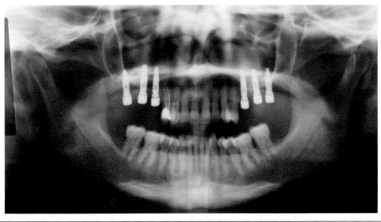

Fig 11-12 z

Fig 11-12 (y, z) Implant placement plus abutment connection was completed five months after the reconstruction.

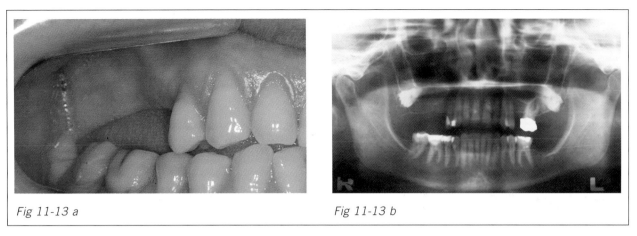

Fig 11-13 a

Fig 11-13 b

Fig 11-13 (a, b) This unilateral edentulous case depicts a narrow ridge combined with a vertical defect at the right posterior maxilla. Even for unilateral cases the proximal tibia constitutes an excellent donor site due to the minimal trauma associated with it.

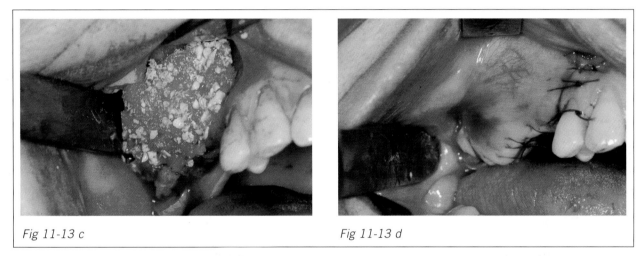

Fig 11-13 c

Fig 11-13 d

Fig 11-13 (c, d) Particulated bone from the tibia mixed with PRP is used to fill the sinus preparation and at the same time to increase the width of the crest. Mixing cancellous bone with PRP aids in achieving primary stability of the veneer. To maintain this lateral reconstruction in place it is essential to avoid the use of a removable denture because of the risk of resorption secondary to pressure.

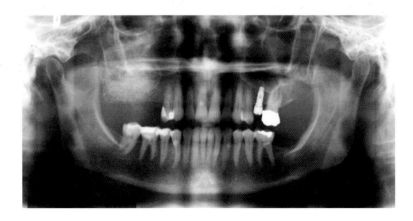

Fig 11-13 (e) Panoramic X-ray after the reconstruction.

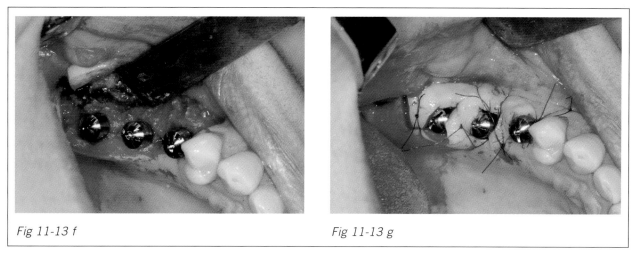

Fig 11-13 f   Fig 11-13 g

Fig 11-13 (f, g) Re-entry five months post-operatively and after 15mm implant placement. Immediate abutment connection can be planned if tailoring of the soft tissues provides sufficient protection of the reconstruction.

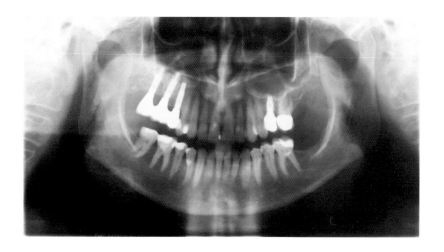

Fig 11-13 (h) Finished case.

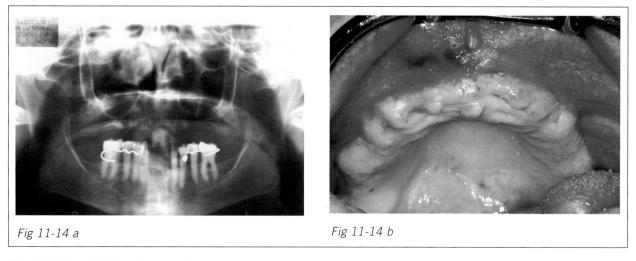

Fig 11-14 a   Fig 11-14 b

Fig 11-14 (a, b) Edentulous maxilla suitable for bilateral sinus lift and implant placement at a second stage.

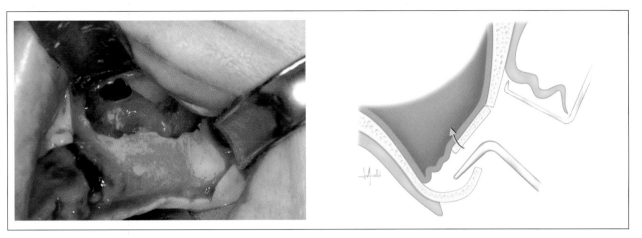

Fig 11-14 (c) When elevating the membrane on the left sinus, a 10mm tear was detected. It is important to bear in mind that particulated materials require the integrity of the membrane to be preserved.

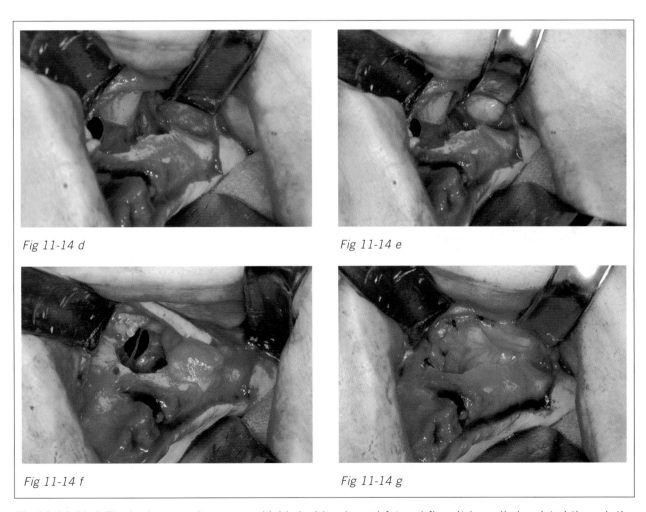

Fig 11-14 d

Fig 11-14 e

Fig 11-14 f

Fig 11-14 g

Fig 11-14 (d-g) The broken membrane was shielded with a buccal fat pad flap. It is easily herniated through the periosteum beneath the zygomatic buttress. Sutured to the anterior part of the window, it recreates a new, well-vascularised roof for the reconstruction.

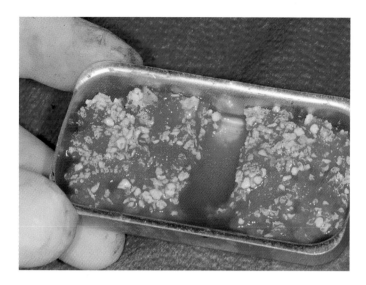

Fig 11-14 (h) Cancellous bone enriched with anorganic matrix and PRP.

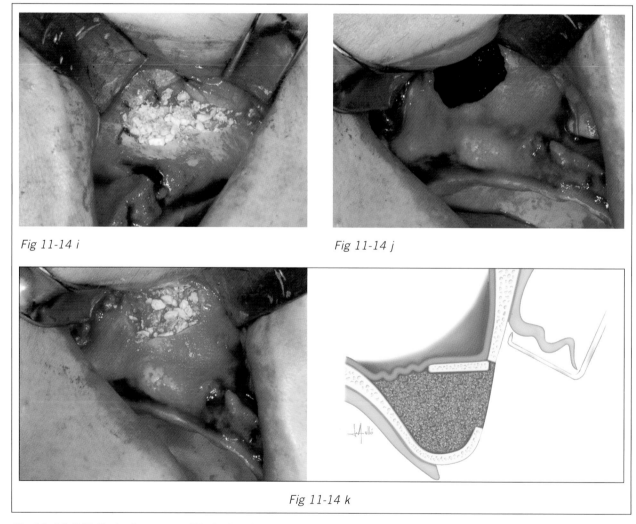

Fig 11-14 i

Fig 11-14 j

Fig 11-14 k

Fig 11-14 (i-k) Both sinuses are filled with the composite graft.

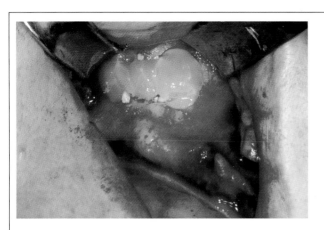

Fig 11-14 l

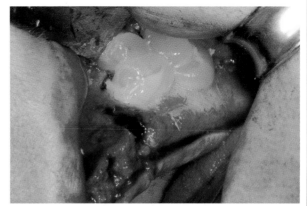

Fig 11-14 m

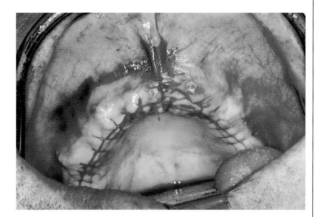

Fig 11-14 (l-n) A portion of PRP is used as a membrane to further protect the reconstruction before a watertight closure.

Fig 11-14 n

229

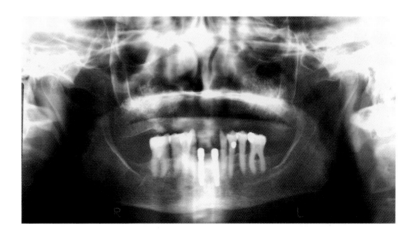

Fig 11-14 (o) Control panoramic X-ray.

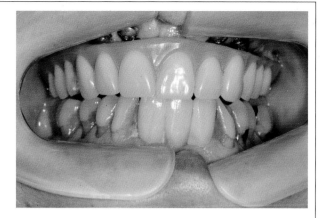

Fig 11-14 p

Fig 11-14 q

Fig 11-14 (p, q) Four months after primary surgery, ten 18mm fixtures were placed and adequate primary stability allowed immediate loading of the posterior six fixtures.

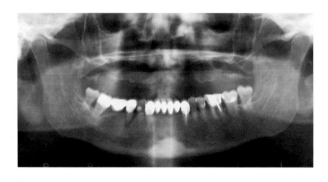

Fig 11-15 (a) Bilateral vertical atrophy associated with a narrow ridge in the anterior maxilla.

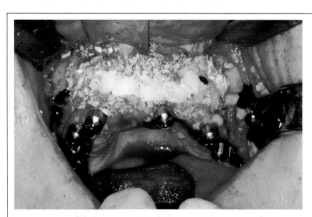

Fig 11-15 b

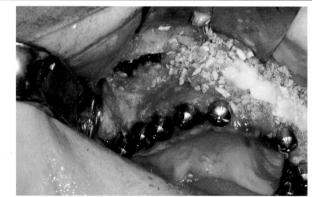

Fig 11-15 c

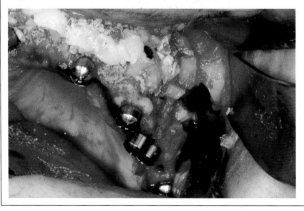

Fig 11-15 d

Fig 11-15 (b-d) Bilateral sinus reconstruction is associated with onlay grafting of the tibia plus PRP and anorganic matrix to improve AP projection. Note how plasma helps to adhere the graft to the recipient site in a veneer fashion. Fixture placement is achieved at the same time.

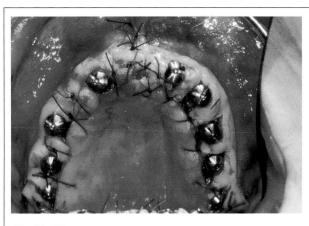

Fig 11-15 e

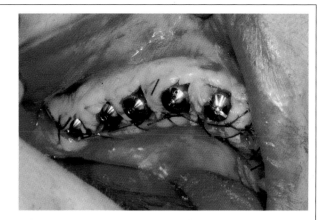

Fig 11-15 f

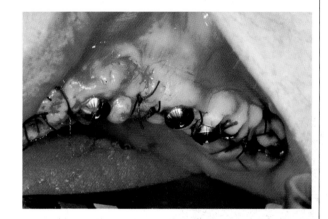

Fig 11-15 (e-g) Primary closure after abutment connection is achieved by creating miniflaps to aid in papilla reconstruction.

Fig 11-15 g

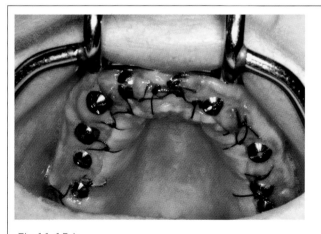

Fig 11-15 h

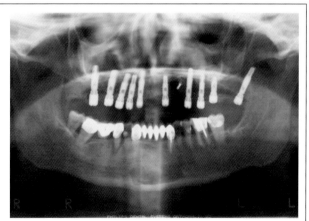

Fig 11-15 i

Fig 11-15 (h, I) Control one week after the procedure.

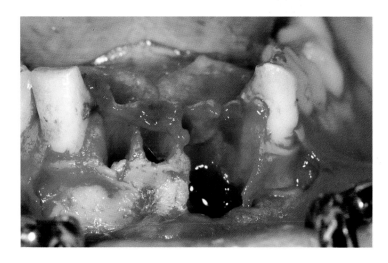

Fig 11-16 (a) Moderate bony defect created after removal of anterior mandibular teeth with endo-perio problems

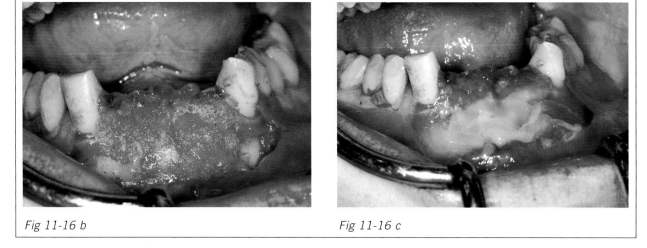

Fig 11-16 b   *Fig 11-16 c*

Fig 11-16 (b, c) Reconstruction of the defective zone is achieved with tibia bone graft and PRP.

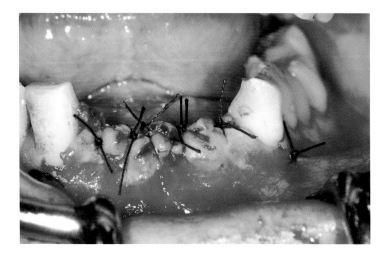

Fig 11-16 (d) Watertight closure

References

1   O'Keefe RM, Reimer BL, Butterfield SL. Harvesting of autogenous cancellous bone graft from the proximal tibia metaphysis: A review of 230 cases. J Orthop Trauma 1991;5:469.

2   Catone GA, Reimer BL, McNeir D, et al. Tibial autogenous cancellous bone as an alternative donor site in maxillofacial surgery: A preliminary report. J Oral Maxillofac Surg 1992;50:1258.

3   Ilankovan V, Stronczek M, Telfer M, et al. A prospective study of trephined bone grafts of the tibial shaft and iliac crest. Br J Oral Maxillofac Surg 1998;36:434.

4   Van Damme PA, Merkx MAV. A modification of the tibial bone graft harvesting technique. Int J Oral Maxillofac Surg 1996;25:246.

5   Besly W, Ward-Booth P. Technique for harvesting tibial cancellous bone modified for use in children. Br J Oral Maxillofac Surg 1999;37:129.

6   Silva RG. Donor site morbidity and patient satisfaction after harvesting iliac and tibial bone. J Oral Maxillofac Surg 1996;54:28.

7   Marchena JM, Block MS, Stover JD. Tibial bone harvesting under intravenous sedation: Morbidity and patient experiences. J Oral Maxillofac Surg 2002;60:1151.

8   Herford AS, Brett JK, Audia F, Becktor J. Medial approach for tibial bone graft: Anatomic study and clinical technique. J Oral Maxillofac Surg 2003;60:358.

9   Hernández Alfaro F, Martí C, Biosca MJ, Gimeno J. Minimally invasive tibial bone harvesting under intravenous sedation. J Oral Maxillofac Surg 2005;63:464.

233